Techniques in Life Science and Biomedicine for the Non-Expert

Series editor

Alexander E. Kalyuzhny, University of Minnesota, Minneapolis, MN, USA

The goal of this series is to provide concise but thorough introductory guides to various scientific techniques, aimed at both the non-expert researcher and novice scientist. Each book will highlight the advantages and limitations of the technique being covered, identify the experiments to which the technique is best suited, and include numerous figures to help better illustrate and explain the technique to the reader. Currently, there is an abundance of books and journals offering various scientific techniques to experts, but these resources, written in technical scientific jargon, can be difficult for the non-expert, whether an experienced scientist from a different discipline or a new researcher, to understand and follow. These techniques, however, may in fact be quite useful to the non-expert due to the interdisciplinary nature of numerous disciplines, and the lack of sufficient comprehensible guides to such techniques can and does slow down research and lead to employing inadequate techniques, resulting in inaccurate data. This series sets out to fill the gap in this much needed scientific resource.

More information about this series at http://www.springer.com/series/13601

Rowa Yousef Alhabbab

Basic Serological Testing

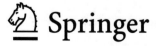 Springer

Rowa Yousef Alhabbab
Division of Applied Medical Sciences and Infectious Disease Unit
King Fahad Centre for Medical Research
King Abdulaziz University
Jeddah, Saudi Arabia

ISSN 2367-1114   ISSN 2367-1122   (electronic)
Techniques in Life Science and Biomedicine for the Non-Expert
ISBN 978-3-030-08515-5   ISBN 978-3-319-77694-1   (eBook)
https://doi.org/10.1007/978-3-319-77694-1

Printed on acid-free paper

This Springer imprint is published by the registered company Springer International Publishing AG part
of Springer Nature.
The registered company address is: Gewerbestrasse 11, 6330 Cham, Switzerland

Foreword

There is only one good, knowledge, and one evil, ignorance.

Socrates

I am pleased to write a foreword to *Basic Serological Testing*, an excellent immunology book written by Rowa Yousef Alhabbab. Drawing upon my experience of more than 30 years as a researcher and 15 years as a book editor, I wish to say without any hesitation that this is a well-written and much-needed book – not only for students who specialize in clinical immunology, but also for learners and seasoned researchers from other disciplines who are interested in finding a concise introductory course on serological testing.

In this book, the author clearly explains the terminology, goals, and clinical workflow of serological testing. There are 16 chapters that walk the reader through the complexities and challenges of serological testing in a step-by-step approach. The main objective of the book is to make complicated and difficult subjects easy to understand and memorize. The book is packed with excellent illustrations and descriptions outlining the main concepts and clarifying the bits and pieces that comprise serological testing. Each chapter includes a "Study Questions" section aimed at improving the learning process and increasing comprehension of the educational material.

I would not be surprised to see this book on the "radar" of creative teachers, whose courses will benefit from incorporating many of the ideas in the book into their classroom instructional materials.

Creating resources for the use of students, teachers, and experienced scientists is a noble but extremely challenging task. Therefore, I wish to express my appreciation to the author, who has shown herself to be a talented and creative teacher who has done a great job converting her expertise into an eloquent and timely educational resource. It could even be considered a back-pocket guide to serological testing techniques.

Understanding scientific principles and methodologies is the key to new knowledge, and if we wish to succeed in our endeavors, we have no alternative but to educate ourselves. The ability to gain new knowledge is critical for successfully advancing science and technology. But success is not always guaranteed and does not come easily: it requires persistence and dedication.

This eloquent book will therefore help to facilitate the acquisition of new knowledge, making our mission possible.

University of Minnesota   Alexander E. Kalyuzhny
Minneapolis, MN, USA

Preface

This book has been written to meet the technical information needs of students in medical laboratories. The first chapter is devoted to a general introduction to the immune system, followed by a chapter clarifying the relationship between antigens and antibodies, in addition to the most common dilution methods used in both clinical and research laboratories, and general safety rules for working in laboratories. The rest of the book addresses the aims, principles, materials, methodologies, and interpretation of the results of the major serological tests that are used during research or in clinical laboratories.

This book is supported with diagrams and colored figures to increase user friendliness and facilitate the study process for students.

Jeddah, Saudi Arabia   Rowa Yousef Alhabbab

Acknowledgements

I would like to express my gratitude to my amazing family for all their support and help, especially my parents, who have supported me throughout my life and have given me everything that has made me what I am today; my wonderful sisters and my beautiful niece and especially my star nephew, Yousef Khouqeer, for his great support.

Moreover, I would like to express my appreciation to all my in-laws for their continuous support, encouragement, and understanding while I wrote this book, particularly my husband, Fahd Abo-ouf. Also, I would like to thank my two children, Saud and Joanna, for their existence in my life and for making the writing process so smooth.

Furthermore, I would like to thank Prof. Esam Azhar for providing me with a remarkable space and environment for writing this book and for all his support along the way. Special thanks go to the staff of Springer, in particular Rita Beck, and the amazing editor, Alexander Kalyuzhny, who helped with the publication of this book.

Contents

1 Introduction to the Immune System 1

Innate Immunity 2

    Physical and Chemical Barriers 2

    Cells of the Innate Immune System 2

    Complement 3

Adaptive Immunity 4

    Clonal Selection Theory 4

    Active, Passive, and Adoptive Immunization 5

    Characteristics of the Adaptive Immune System 6

    Cells Involved in the Adaptive Immune System................ 6

    The Cellular and Humoral Adaptive Immune System 7

References... 8

Study Questions 9

2 Antibody and Antigen Interaction 15

Antigens 15

    Antigen Foreignness..................................... 16

    Antigen Molecular Weight 16

    Antigen Chemical Complexity 16

    Antigen and MHC Molecules.............................. 16

Antibodies.. 17

Interaction of Antibodies and Antigens 17

Dilutions 18

    $C_1 V_1 = C_2 V_2$ Method................................. 18

    Dilution Factor Method................................... 18

    Serial Dilution.. 19

General Safety Rules for Clinical Laboratories 19

References.. 21

Study Questions 21

3 Precipitation and Agglutination Reactions. 23
  Precipitation Technique. 24
    Principle 24
  Agglutination 26
    Principle 26
    Application 28
  Hemagglutination 28
    Principle 28
    Application 29
  References. 30
  Study Questions 30

4 Rapid Plasma Reagin (RPR) Test 31
  Rapid Plasma Reagin (RPR) Test 32
    Principle 32
    RPR Test Reagents 32
    RPR Test Steps 33
  References. 33
  Study Questions 34

5 *Treponema pallidum* Hemagglutination (TPHA) Test 35
  Treponema Pallidum Hemagglutination (TPHA) Test 36
    Principle 36
    Reagents That Must Be Provided in the Kit 36
    TPHA Test Steps. 36
    Results Interpretation 37
  References. 38
  Study Questions 38

6 Stained *Brucella* Suspensions. 41
  The Most Pathogenic *Brucella* Species to Humans 42
    Brucella abortus 42
    Brucella melitensis 42
    Brucella suis 42
  Brucellosis Incubation Period. 43
  Serological Tests to Detect Brucellosis. 43
  Slide Agglutination Test 43
    Principle 43
    Reagents 44
    Steps 44
  Serum Agglutination Test, Tube (SAT). 44
    Principle 44
    Reagents 45
    SAT Test Steps 45
    Results Interpretation 45
  References. 46
  Study Questions 47

7 Rheumatoid Factor (RF) 49
   RF Latex Agglutination Test.................................... 50
      Principle 50
      The Application of the RF Latex Agglutination Test 50
      Reagents and Materials Used 50
      RF Latex Agglutination Test Steps 51
      Results Interpretation 51
      RF Latex Agglutination Test Limitations 51
   References.. 51
   Study Questions 52

8 Suspension Anti-Streptolysin-O (ASO/ASL) Test 55
   ASO/ASL Test 56
      Principle 56
      ASO/ASL Test Application.................................. 56
      ASO/ASL Test Reagents.................................... 56
      ASO/ASL Test Steps....................................... 56
      Results Interpretation 57
   References.. 57
   Study Questions 58

9 C-Reactive Protein (CRP) Latex Agglutination Test 59
   CRP Latex Agglutination Test 60
      Principle 60
      Applications and Significance................................ 60
      Reagents 60
      Test Steps 60
      Results Interpretation 61
   References.. 61
   Study Questions 62

10 Complement Fixation Test (CFT) 63
   Complement Fixation Test 63
      Principle 63
      Reagents Provided in the Kit 64
      Preparation of CFT Reagents 64
      Preparation of Complement and Sensitized sRBCs 65
      Standard Antigen Preparation............................... 67
      Positive Control and Antisera Preparation 70
      CFT Steps 72
      Results Interpretation 72
   Reference 74
   Study Questions 74

11 Radioimmunoassay (RIA) 77
   Radioimmunoassay (RIA) 77
      Principle 77
      RIA Reagents 78
      RIA Steps 78
      RIA Results Interpretation 80
   References... 81
   Study Questions 81

**12 Enzyme Immunoassay (EIAs) and Enzyme-Linked
    Immunosorbent Assay (ELISA)**............................. 83
   Enzyme-Linked Immunosorbent Assay (ELISA).................. 83
      Principle 83
      ELISA Reagents and Steps................................ 88
      ELISA Results Interpretation 92
   References... 93
   Study Questions 93

13 Pregnancy Test... 97
   HCG One-Step Pregnancy Urine Test Device 98
      Principle 98
      Reagents 98
      Steps 98
      Results Interpretation 99
   References... 100
   Study Questions 102

14 Radial Immunodiffusion (RID) 105
   Radial Immunodiffusion (RID) Assay 105
      Principle 105
      Reagents 107
      Steps 107
      Results Interpretation 107
   References... 108
   Study Questions 109

15 Immunofixation Electrophoresis (IFE) 111
   Immunofixation Electrophoresis............................... 112
      Principle 112
      Reagents 112
      Steps 114
      Results Interpretation 115
   References... 116
   Study Questions 117

16 Immunofluorescence (IF) Assay 119
     Immunofluorescence (IF) Assay 119
        Principle 119
        Reagents 122
        Steps 124
        Results Interpretation 125
     References 125
     Study Questions 125

Glossary 127

Index 135

Chapter 1
Introduction to the Immune System

Learning Objectives
By the end of this chapter the reader should be able to:

1. Understand the functions of the immune system.
2. Describe the role and importance of each line of defense in the immune system.
3. Understand the functions and components of the physical and the chemical barriers.
4. State the key players and describe the function of the cellular innate immunity.
5. Understand the complement system.
6. Explain the clonal expansion theory.
7. Differentiate between the types of immunization.
8. Describe the features of the adaptive immune system.
9. Define and explain the function of cellular and humoral adaptive immunity.

The main function of the immune system is to defend the host and maintain **homeostasis**. Any dysregulation in the immune system can lead to several immunological diseases such as **autoimmune disorders**, cancer, or chronic inflammation. Luckily, the immune system is sophisticated enough to regulate itself to maintain the behavior of its cellular components to interact with foreign particles, producing protective responses. A major characteristic of a healthy immune system is its ability to remember and recognize pathogens years after the initial exposure. This form of memory relies heavily on the ability to distinguish self- and non-self-antigens. The ability of the immune system to differentiate between host tissue and foreign particles such as pathogens relies mainly on cell surface molecules that are capable of recognizing, binding, and adhering to other molecules in a specific manner. The different ways in which the body responds to foreign pathogens fall into two main categories of defense that divide the immune system into **innate** and **adaptive immunity**.

© Springer International Publishing AG, part of Springer Nature 2018
R. Y. Alhabbab, *Basic Serological Testing*, Techniques in Life Science and Biomedicine for the Non-Expert, https://doi.org/10.1007/978-3-319-77694-1_1

Innate Immunity

The innate immune system consists of cells and several elements that are always available to protect the host from any foreign pathogens in a short time. Innate immunity includes all body surfaces and several internal components, such as the mucous membrane and the cough reflex. Moreover, innate immunity includes chemical barriers such as stomach acidity and pH. Other components of the innate immune system include the **complement system** and many other features such as fever, **interferon**, and cell receptors such as **pattern recognition receptors (PRRs)** [1, 2]. The cellular arm of the innate immune system includes **phagocytic cells** such as dendritic cells (DCs), macrophages/monocytes, and neutrophils. Several other cells are also considered to be innate immune cells such as **natural killer (NK) cells** and **platelets**.

Physical and Chemical Barriers

For microorganisms to interact with the cells of the innate immune system, they have to penetrate and pass through the host physical and chemical barriers. The most important physical barrier that microbes have to penetrate to enter the host body is the skin [3]. Although some pathogens can gain access via sebaceous glands and hair follicles, the presence of several chemical molecules such as acidic sweat, sebaceous secretions, fatty acids, and hydrolytic enzymes provide protection against the invading pathogens, minimizing the significance of this path of infection [4]. The respiratory and gastrointestinal tracts can serve as two important gates for pathogens; therefore, the innate immune system has provided these two areas with several mechanisms that can give initial protection against pathogens. For instance, the mucous membrane, which covers these areas, can trap the pathogens that would subsequently be swept toward the external opening by ciliated epithelial cells [3, 4]. Additional mechanisms that the innate immune system provides to protect the respiratory tract are nasal hair and the cough reflex. Several factors can play a key role in protecting the gastrointestinal tract, including the low pH of the stomach, saliva hydrolytic enzymes, and proteolytic enzyme and bile of the small intestine [4].

Cells of the Innate Immune System

As mentioned earlier, the cellular components of the innate immune system includes monocytes/macrophages, neutrophils, DCs, basophils, eosinophils, and platelets.

Basophils, eosinophils, and neutrophils are considered to be **polymorphonuclear (PMN)** cells, which are also known as **granulocytes**. These cells are characterized as short-lived phagocytic cells, and contain several enzymic and toxic molecules capable of destroying some microorganisms [5]. The important role that PMNs play in the immune system appears when they are defective, which is usually associated with recurrent and chronic infections [4]. Blood-circulating monocytes once residing in tissue, differentiate into macrophages. Macrophages are long-lived phagocytic cells that contain many degradative particles to process the phagocytized pathogens that would subsequently be presented on their surface to antigen-specific T cells [6]. Therefore, macrophages are phagocytic and **antigen-presenting cells (APCs)** [7]. However, DCs are considered to be the most crucial APCs of the innate immune system because of their ability to migrate after phagocytizing the pathogen from the site of infection to the **secondary lymphoid organs**, where they trigger the adaptive immune responses with very high efficiency [4].

Virally infected and cancer cells have abnormally altered membranes that are distinguished by NK cells [8]. NK cells release very powerful intracellular molecules upon contact with their target cells leading to pore formation and the lysis of the target cells [8]. Therefore, NK cells are considered to be **cytotoxic cells** [8].

Generally, most of the innate immune cells recognize conserved structures in pathogens known as **pathogen-associated molecular patterns (PAMPs)** [9]. PAMPs are recognized by several families of receptors known as PRRs, such as toll-like receptors (TLRs), C-type lectin receptors (CLRs), NOD-like receptors , and RIG-like receptors [4, 10]. Some of these receptors are expressed extracellularly, whereas some are expressed intracellularly, and each recognizes and binds to specific PAMPs [9]. For instance, TLR-9 is expressed intracellularly and recognizes viral and bacterial DNA, whereas TLR-4 is expressed extracellularly and identifies **lipopolysaccharide (LPS)** in Gram-negative and some Gram-positive bacteria [4, 9].

Complement

Complement is an important component of the innate immune system, and consists of about 25 proteins that are produced via the hepatocytes of the liver [4]. Complement circulates in the body in its inactive form, and can be activated through three pathways: **classical**, **alternative**, and **lectin**. The first protein of the classical pathway (**C1q**) is activated in response to antibody-antigen particles; therefore, the classical pathway participates in the adaptive immune system [11]. Unlike the classical pathway, which requires antibody-antigen particles, the alternative pathway becomes activated directly through the binding of **C3** to the surface of a pathogen [11–13]. Lectin pathway activation involves the binding of **C2** and **C4** to mannan moieties on the surface of pathogens [11, 12]. Regardless of the pathway that has activated the complement system, all three pathways initiate a chain of events leading to the eventual formation of the **membrane attack complex (MAC),** which results in the lysis of the pathogens [4].

Some complement components can coat (**opsonize**) the pathogen directly to facilitate the process of phagocytosis [12]. Phagocytic cells express complement receptors that facilitate their binding to complement opsonizing pathogens.

Table 1.1 The components of the complement system pathways and their functions

	Classical pathway	Alternative pathway	Lectin pathway
First activated complement component	C1q	C3	MBP (mannan-binding protein)
Complement system functions	Opsonization	Inflammation mediators	MAC formation and cell lysis
Complement component involved	C3b	C4b	C5b
		C3a	C6
		C5a	C7
			C8
			C9

Moreover, upon complement activation, some complement components are released to recruit various cells of the immune system to the site of invasion. Table 1.1 summarizes the components of the complement system pathways and their functions.

Adaptive Immunity

The response of the adaptive immune system comes relatively late, days to weeks after exposure to pathogens. Similar to the innate immunity, the adaptive immune system consists of cellular and non-cellular (also called humoral) components. Cell-mediated adaptive immunity achieved by T and B lymphocytes. Specific antigen activation of **T** and **B cells** directly or indirectly involves APCs such as DCs, where their interaction with lymphocytes leads to the proliferation and differentiation of lymphocytes into effector T and B cells that mediate cellular and **humoral responses** [4]. Cells of the adaptive immune system are characterized by their ability to clonally expand, the theory that explains this phenomenon is called **clonal selection theory** [4]. This process provides the host with mounting numbers of antigen-specific cells that can respond rapidly to the same antigen in the future, a process known as **memory** [14].

Any compound that can induce adaptive immune responses is called an **antigen**. This term comes from the ability of these compounds to lead to the generation of **antibodies** [4]. However, antigens are also compounds that have the ability to generate antibody-mediated and T-cell-mediated immune responses.

Clonal Selection Theory

The specificity of the immune system is a feature that comes from the ability of B and T cells to recognize and bind only to their specific antigens and respond to eliminate them. The **clonal expansion** of T and B cells is very complicated; however, some errors or mutations may occasionally occur, leading to the generation of receptors not specific or poorly specific to the target antigen, or in the worst case, autoreactive [4]. Normally, non-functional cells are terminated, but in some cases they survive without any associated harm [4]. Nevertheless, autoreactively generated cells are either suppressed by regulatory immune cells such as **regulatory T (Treg) cells** or are **clonally deleted** [15]. The survival and the release of these autoreactive cells may lead to continuous autoimmune responses. During lymphocyte development, self-reactive lymphocytes are also eliminated or inactivated [4].

The proposal of the clonal selection theory includes the following:

1. The immune system builds mounting numbers of T and B cells with various specificities before contacting their foreign-specific antigens [14, 16].
2. Lymphocyte-specific receptors , which are activated via their target antigens, release different products [16]. For example, B cells possess specific antigen receptors on their surface known as **B cell receptors (BCRs)**. The binding of this receptor to its specific antigen leads to B cell activation and differentiation into plasma cells, which eventually produce antibodies specific to that antigen, whereas T cell--specific receptors are called **T cell receptors (TCRs)** that, upon binding to their specific antigen, become activated to produce several products such as **cytokines**, which are proteins produced to help in the elimination of pathogens by guiding the immune cell responses [17–19].
3. Each single lymphocyte has its own specific cell receptor that has only single specificity to one particular antigen [16]. The invading pathogen selects and binds to its specific TCRs and BCRs expressed on lymphocytes from all the available receptors [18, 19].

The remainder of the clonal selection theory proposal is to explain the process of antigen selection from the various repertoires of the available receptors, as follows:

1. The binding of lymphocyte cell surface receptors to their specific antigens or part of it called **epitope** leads to their activation, proliferation, and differentiation into clones of cells with receptors of the same specificity for the initial corresponding antigen [4].
2. Activated B cells produce antibodies specific to the corresponding antigen. Similarly, activated T cells proliferate and generate a clone of cells with the same specificity, and produce several cytokines, which results in the activation of many cells [4].

The final result is the generation of several different clones of B and T cells producing specific antibodies and cytokines respectively.

Active, Passive, and Adoptive Immunization

Immunization can induce adaptive immunity in several ways:

1. **Active immunization**: this type of immunity is achieved by the administration of the target antigen to an individual [4].
2. **Passive immunization**: transferring specific antibodies generated in an immunized individual to non-immunized persons [4].
3. **Adoptive immunization**: this kind of immunization involves the transfer of immune cells to non-immunized individuals [4].

Characteristics of the Adaptive Immune System

Generally, the adaptive immune system is distinguished from other systems in the host, such as the respiratory system, circulation, and reproduction by common and unique features that are listed below:

1. The adaptive immune system has the capability to recognize and respond to various, specific, and unique molecular entities when needed. Therefore, the response mediated by the adaptive immune system is not a random or undifferentiated response, but specific [18, 19].
2. The adaptive immune system can respond to new, previously unseen molecules, a characteristic known as adaptiveness.
3. The adaptive immune system has the ability to discriminate between self- and non-self-antigens [19].
4. The adaptive immune system can remember previously encountered foreign molecules and initiate a faster and stronger response than the first response to the same molecule, a characteristic known as memory or anamnestic response [14].

Cells Involved in the Adaptive Immune System

The cellular arm of the adaptive immune system is composed of two types of lymphocytes, namely B and T lymphocytes. Generally, lymphocytes are derived from a common lymphoid precursor cell; however, B cell developmental stages take place in the bone marrow, whereas T cell precursors are released from the bone marrow and then mature in the thymus [20]. APCs participate in adaptive immune responses through their direct interaction with T cells. The family of APCs consists mainly of macrophages and DCs. These cells, unlike lymphocytes, do not express antigen-specific receptors; rather, they express different molecules on their surface that facilitate their interactions with T cells [19]. The most important molecules expressed on the surface of APCs are **major histocompatibility complex (MHC)** molecules. MHC molecules are divided into two major classes, MHC class I and class II. Each class interacts strictly with one of the T cell subsets. For example,

MHC class I interacts with CD8 T cells, whereas MHC class II interacts with CD4 T cells. In humans, MHC molecules are encoded by two sets of polymorphic genes expressed on chromosome 6 [4]. The major function of APCs is to phagocytize pathogen or foreign particles, process the ingested protein antigens, locate various peptides from the processed antigen non-covalently to MHC molecules, and display it on their surface for T cells [18, 19]. The display of peptide-MHC complexes on the surface subsequently results in T cell activation.

The Cellular and Humoral Adaptive Immune System

Immune responses mediated by the adaptive immune system is mainly divided into humoral (B cells mediated) and cellular responses (mediated by T cells).

Humoral Immunity

B cell receptor-activated B cells produce antibodies specific to the antigen that have initially activated the B cells through its BCR, which is a membrane antigen-specific immunoglobulin (Ig) molecule. Each B cell has been estimated to express about 100,000 BCRs of an individual specificity [21]. A serum contains a heterogeneous mixture of globulins specific to a single antigen, immunoglobulin is a term that refers to serum globulin that possesses antibody activity [4]. Antibodies recognize and bind to specific regions on antigens, known as epitopes to facilitate the phago-cytosis of antigens by **Fc receptors** expressed on APCs [4]. Generally, antibodies consist of two identical heavy (H) and light (L) chains connected through disulfide bridges. Antibodies are divided mainly into two regions fragment antigen-binding (**Fab**) and fragment crystallizable (**Fc**) **regions**. The Fab region is the antigen binding site, and consists of two identical binding regions that bind to two epitopes of the same specificity on the same antigen or on different molecules. Antibodies are also classified into five isotypes called **IgG**, **IgM**, **IgA**, **IgE** and **IgD** according to the differences found in their H chain [21]. Although all antibody classes share a common feature (antigen-binding region), each antibody class has unique functional properties. For example, IgG is the only antibody that can pass through the placenta, whereas IgA is the most abundant antibody in secretions. Antibody–antigen interaction is not covalent, but involves several weak forces, including hydrogen bonds, Van der Waal's forces, and hydrophobic interactions [4]. Because these forces are weak, several factors influence the strength of the antigen–antibody binding such as the size, the charge, and the shape of both the antigen and the antibody binding site [4].

Cell-Mediated Immunity

Cell-mediated immunity is mainly performed by T cells; however, other cells that belong to the innate immune system can also be involved, such as phagocytic cells. Each T cell expresses about 100,000 TCRs of the same specificity that interact directly with the MHC molecules expressed on APCs to produce cytokines [18]. T cells are divided into several populations according to their functions, in particular, the profile of cytokines that they produce and their surface markers. The major two populations of the T cells include **CD4$^+$ T cells (T helper (Th) cells)** and **CD8$^+$ T cells (cytotoxic T (Tc) cells)**. CD4$^+$ T cells are divided into subpopulations according to their cytokine profiles: **Th1, Th2, Th17, T follicular helper (T$_{Fh}$),** and CD4$^+$CD25$^+$ regulatory T (Treg) cells. The main functions performed by T cells are categorized as follows:

1. **Inflammatory role**: CD4$^+$Th1 and Th17, upon activation they produce a variety of cytokines that can induce inflammation via stimulating macrophages and monocytes.
2. **Regulatory function**: CD4$^+$CD25$^+$ Tregs and in some cases Th2, when activated they produce regulatory cytokines that can suppress inflammation such as interleukin-10 (IL-10) [15].
3. **B cell help**: CD4$^+$T$_{Fh}$ cells provide B cells with several signals that are essential for B cell activation and antibody production.
4. **Cytotoxic function**: CD8$^+$T cells are cytotoxic killer T cells [14].
5. **Cytokine production**: T cells, particularly Th cells, communicate with other cells of lymphoid and non-lymphoid origin, directly and indirectly through their cytokines [4].

T cell activation requires two essential signals. The first signal arrives from the interaction between T cell TCRs and the appropriate MHC molecules on APCs. The second signal involves co-stimulators such as the interaction of CD40 on APCs with CD40 ligand on T cells; this signal also includes the involvement of cytokines [4].

Healthy immunity requires the interaction of humoral and cellular components of the adaptive and the innate immune system to eliminate any pathogens.

References

1. Janeway CA Jr, Medzhitov R. Innate immune recognition. Annu Rev Immunol. 2002;20:197–216.
2. Suresh R, Mosser DM. Pattern recognition receptors in innate immunity, host defense, and immunopathology. Adv Physiol Educ. 2013;37(4):281–91.
3. Turvey SE, Broide DH. Innate immunity. J Allergy Clin Immunol. 2010;125(2 Suppl 2):S24–32.
4. Coico R, Sunshine G. Immunology: a short course. 7th ed. Chichester, West Sussex; Hoboken, NJ: John Wiley & Sons Inc.; 2015.
5. Gordon S. Phagocytosis: an immunobiologic process. Immunity. 2016;44(3):463–75.

6. Aderem A, Underhill DM. Mechanisms of phagocytosis in macrophages. Annu Rev Immunol. 1999;17:593–623.
7. Hume DA. Macrophages as APC and the dendritic cell myth. J Immunol. 2008;181(9):5829–35.
8. Hazeldine J, Lord JM. The impact of ageing on natural killer cell function and potential consequences for health in older adults. Ageing Res Rev. 2013;12(4):1069–78.
9. Akira S, Takeda K, Kaisho T. Toll-like receptors: critical proteins linking innate and acquired immunity. Nat Immunol. 2001;2(8):675–80.
10. Mogensen TH. Pathogen recognition and inflammatory signaling in innate immune defenses. Clin Microbiol Rev. 2009;22(2):240–73. Table of Contents.
11. Ricklin D, Lambris JD. Complement in immune and inflammatory disorders: pathophysiological mechanisms. J Immunol. 2013;190(8):3831–8.
12. Carroll MC, Isenman DE. Regulation of humoral immunity by complement. Immunity. 2012;37(2):199–207.
13. Nilsson B, Nilsson EK. The tick-over theory revisited: is C3 a contact-activated protein? Immunobiology. 2012;217(11):1106–10.
14. Amsen D, Backer RA, Helbig C. Decisions on the road to memory. Adv Exp Med Biol. 2013;785:107–20.
15. Ohkura N, Kitagawa Y, Sakaguchi S. Development and maintenance of regulatory T cells. Immunity. 2013;38(3):414–23.
16. Silverstein AM. The clonal selection theory: what it really is and why modern challenges are misplaced. Nat Immunol. 2002;3(9):793–6.
17. Boehm T, Bleul CC. The evolutionary history of lymphoid organs. Nat Immunol. 2007;8(2):131–5.
18. Birnbaum ME, Dong S, Garcia KC. Diversity-oriented approaches for interrogating T-cell receptor repertoire, ligand recognition, and function. Immunol Rev. 2012;250(1):82–101.
19. Brownlie RJ, Zamoyska R. T cell receptor signalling networks: branched, diversified and bounded. Nat Rev Immunol. 2013;13(4):257–69.
20. Blom B, Spits H. Development of human lymphoid cells. Annu Rev Immunol. 2006;24:287–320.
21. Yang J, Reth M. Receptor dissociation and B-cell activation. Curr Top Microbiol Immunol. 2016;393:27–43.

Study Questions

1. **The innate immune system consists of several components such as:**

   (a) Body surfaces.
   (b) Chemical barriers.
   (c) Complement system.
   (d) **All the above.**

2. **The innate cellular immune system includes:**

   (a) T cells.
   (b) B cells.
   (c) **Neutrophils.**
   (d) None of the above.

3. **The first line/s of defense that microorganisms must penetrate before their interaction with the innate immune system is/are:**

   (a) **Physical and chemical barriers of the host.**
   (b) Adaptive immune system.
   (c) Specific immunity.
   (d) Antibodies.

4. **Pathogens that gain access to the respiratory tract can initially be:**

   (a) Killed by the acidity of the area.
   (b) **Swept by ciliated epithelial cells.**
   (c) Destroyed by platelets.
   (d) Damaged by the bile of the tract.

5. **Polymorphonuclear cells of the innate immune system include:**

   (a) B and T cells.
   (b) Platelets.
   (c) Macrophages.
   (d) **Basophils, neutrophils, and eosinophils.**

6. **Polymorphonuclear cells are:**

   (a) **Short-lived phagocytic cells.**
   (b) Long-lived phagocytic cells.
   (c) Cells that, once they reside in the tissue, they differentiate into macrophages.
   (d) Cells that do not contain enzymic and toxic molecules.

7. **Macrophages are:**

   (a) Long-lived phagocytic cells.
   (b) Antigen-presenting cells (APCs).
   (c) Cells that contain degradative particles.
   (d) **All the above.**

8. **The most powerful APCs for pathogens of first-time exposure are:**

   (a) Macrophages.
   (b) Neutrophils.
   (c) B cells.
   (d) **Dendritic cells (DCs).**

9. **The cytotoxic cells of the innate immune system are:**

   (a) Macrophages.
   (b) **NK cells.**
   (c) Neutrophils.
   (d) DCs.

10. **Pathogen-associated molecular patterns (PAMPs) are:**

    (a) Immune cell receptors.
    (b) Conserved structures on host cells.
    (c) **Conserved structures on the pathogens.**
    (d) Not recognizable by any of the immune cell receptors.

11. **Pattern recognition receptors (PRRs) are:**

    (a) Receptors that recognize PAMPs.
    (b) A family of receptors that includes TLRs.
    (c) Expressed by the cells of the innate immune system.
    (d) **All the above.**

12. **PRRs include:**

    (a) B cell receptors (BCRs).
    (b) T cell receptors (TCRs).
    (c) **NOD-like receptors.**
    (d) Complement receptors.

13. **TLR-9 is:**

    (a) **An intracellular receptor.**
    (b) An extracellular receptor.
    (c) A receptor that recognizes the bacterial cell wall.
    (d) A receptor that recognizes the fungal cell membrane.

14. **Complements:**

    (a) Consist of proteins.
    (b) Circulate in the body in their inactive form.
    (c) Synthesize in the liver.
    (d) **All the above.**

15. **Complement activation through the classical pathway requires:**

    (a) **Antibodies---antigens particles**
    (b) The direct binding of C3 to the surface of the pathogens.
    (c) The binding to mannan moieties.
    (d) T cell activation.

16. **Complement functions include:**

    (a) MAC formation.
    (b) Opsonization.
    (c) Inflammation.
    (d) **All the above.**

17. **Cells of the adaptive immune system are characterized by:**

    (a) Their ability to clonally expand.
    (b) Their memory.
    (c) Their specificity.
    (d) **All the above.**

18. **Autoreactive cells can be suppressed by:**

    (a) Neutrophils.
    (b) Interferon.
    (c) **Regulatory T (Treg) cells.**
    (d) Tumor necrosis factor.

19. **The final result of clonal expansion is:**

    (a) The formation of several different clones of cytokines.
    (b) **The formation of several different clones of B and T cells.**
    (c) The formation of several different clones of C-reactive proteins.
    (d) The formation of several different clones of chemokines.

20. **Active immunization is:**

    (a) Immunization that involves the transfer of immune cells.
    (b) Immunization that involves the transfer of specific antibodies.
    (c) **Immunization that involves the administration of target antigen.**
    (d) Immunization that involves the transfer of complements.

21. **T cell activation requires:**

    (a) **Antigen processing and presentation on MHC molecules.**
    (b) Intact antigens.
    (c) B cells activation.
    (d) All the above.

22. **Adaptive humoral immunity is:**

    (a) T cells mediated.
    (b) DCs mediated.
    (c) NKT cells mediated.
    (d) **B cells mediated.**

23. **Cellular adaptive immunity is mainly mediated by:**

    (a) B cells.
    (b) **T cells.**
    (c) NK cells.
    (d) Platelets.

24. **T cell populations and subpopulations include:**

   (a) CD4 T cells and CD8 T cells.
   (b) Th1 and Th2.
   (c) Tregs.
   (d) **All the above.**

25. **T cell functions include:**

   (a) Cytotoxicity.
   (b) Regulatory function.
   (c) B cell help.
   (d) **All the above**

Chapter 2
Antibody and Antigen Interaction

Learning Objectives
By the end of this chapter the reader should be able to:

1. Understand what antigen and immunogen characteristics are.
2. Describe the basic structure of an antibody.
3. Understand the interaction between antigens and their antibodies.
4. Understand how to use the different methods of dilution that are commonly used in serology.
5. Understand the general safety rules for clinical laboratories.

Before discussing in greater detail most of the main serological methods that are being used in clinical immunology laboratories, it is necessary to briefly explain the definitions of antigens, antibodies, and their interactions.

Antigens

Antigens are foreign molecules that can specifically bind to the B cell receptor (BCR) on B cells or soluble antibodies. Antigens that are capable of inducing immune responses are called **immunogens** [1, 2]. Therefore, not all antigens are immunogens, but all immunogens are antigens. For an antigen to be immunogenic, it must have a large molecular weight, chemical complexity, be foreign, and be presented on major histocompatibility complex (MHC) molecules [3].

© Springer International Publishing AG, part of Springer Nature 2018
R. Y. Alhabbab, *Basic Serological Testing*, Techniques in Life Science and
Biomedicine for the Non-Expert, https://doi.org/10.1007/978-3-319-77694-1_2

Antigen Foreignness

Foreignness is the first characteristic required for a compound to be immunogenic. Therefore, the more foreign an antigen is, and the less self-antigen it is, the more immunogenic it is [3].

Antigen Molecular Weight

A substance's molecular weight plays an important role in determining the immunogenicity of a compound. In short, compounds with larger molecular weight are more likely to be immunogenic [3]. For instance, compounds smaller than 1,000 Da are not immunogenic; however, compounds larger than 6,000 Da are usually immunogenic [3].

Antigen Chemical Complexity

Antigen chemical complexity can determine not only whether an antigen is immunogenic, but also the level of its immunogenicity [3]. For example, a compound of 60,000 Da in size consisting of homopolymer amino acid is not immunogenic because it is not chemically complex [3]. Therefore, antigen immunogenicity depends on the compound's chemical complexity, regardless of its molecular weight. Moreover, the more chemically complex compounds are, the more immunogenic they are.

Antigen and MHC Molecules

Antigens can neither be recognized nor activate the T cells directly; therefore, antigens must be processed by antigen-presenting cells (APCs) and express on their surface MHC molecules. Subsequently, T cell receptors (TCR) recognize the antigen specifically via their antigenic epitopes expressed on APC MHC molecules [4, 5]. Antigenic epitopes are the smallest part of an antigen, are recognized by the immune system, and are capable of binding to antibodies and TCRs [6]. The degradation of an antigen protein in nature depends on two key factors: the antigen stability, and antigen susceptibility to degradation by enzymes used by APCs to process the antigen [3]. For example, some peptides can be resistant to enzymic degradation such as D-amino acid peptides; therefore, they are not immunogenic [3].

Antibodies

Antibodies, also known as immunoglobulins, are proteins produced by B cells. They are specific to certain molecules, and can circulate freely. Immunoglobulins are available in two forms: either membrane-bound to the surface of B cells and known as BCR, or in a secreted form. **Plasma cells** are the factory of antibodies and are the final differentiated B cells that mainly reside in the bone marrow [3].

The basic structure of an immunoglobulin consists of two identical polypeptide heavy chains (about 53,000 Da in size) and two identical polypeptide light chains (about 22,000 Da in size) [3]. These polypeptide chains are linked together via several disulfide bonds [7]. Antibodies can also be divided into two fragments, the Fab (fragment antigen-binding) and the Fc (fragment crystallizable) fragments (Fig. 2.1) [3, 7]. The Fab fragment consists of two identical antigen binding sites specific to one antigenic epitope [3]. On the other hand, the Fc region of an antibody is responsible for its biological function following the binding of an antigen to the Fab region of that antibody [7].

The heavy chain of an antibody can then be divided into five classes: IgM, IgG, IgA, IgE, and IgD.

Interaction of Antibodies and Antigens

An antibody is characterized by its specificity to target antigen. This fact serves as the basis of many **serological** assays. Antibody–antigen-specific interaction is used in vitro to identify various microorganisms (**serotyping**). The interaction between an antibody and its multivalent antigen leads to one of three results: **precipitation**, **agglutination**, and complement activation, all of which are discussed later in this book [3]. However, if antigens or antibodies are univalent, none of the above-mentioned results would occur [3]. Therefore, for precipitation, agglutination or complement activation to happen, the antigen in the reaction must be multivalent and the antibody divalent.

Fig. 2.1 Structure of an antibody

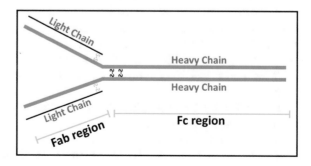

The interaction between antigen and antibody is relatively weak and does not involve any covalent bond [1]. The binding forces involved in the interaction between antibodies and antigens are mainly electrostatic forces, van der Waals forces, and hydrophobic forces [1]. Therefore, antibody–antigen reactions can be easily dissociated by high salt concentration, extreme pH levels, or by chemotropic ions [3]. The strength of the interaction between antibodies and antigens is called **affinity**, whereas the overall binding energy is known as **avidity** [3]. Therefore, IgM avidity is higher than IgG, even if both of them possess the same Fab affinity to their target antigen, and this is mainly because IgM has more binding sites than IgG.

Dilutions

Dilution is an important process that is widely used in clinical and in research laboratories. Therefore, it is critical to explain the most commonly used methods of dilution that are particularly utilized with serological testing.

$C_1V_1 = C_2V_2$ Method

This method is mainly used to prepare a diluted solution from a stock of known concentration. Here, C_1 stands for the concentration of the stock solution, whereas C_2 stands for the final concentration of the newly prepared solution. V_1, on the othe hand, is the required volume from the stock solution to prepare the new one, whereas V_2 is the final volume of the new solution.

Dilution Factor Method

This type of dilution uses the following formula:
   Dilution factor (DF) = final volume/stock volume.
   The latter formula is utlized to dilute a solution without using the stock concentration. This method expresses the solution as a ratio where the stock is a part of the total parts. For instance, a DF of 20 means 1:20 dilution, in other words, one part of stock and 19 parts of diluant results in a total of 20 parts. An additional example includes preparing 1:300 dilution in a total volume of 600 μL, by using the above formula:
   DF (300) = final volume (600 μL)/stock volume
   By rearranging the equation:
   Stock volume = 600 μL/300 = 2 μL
   This means that 2 μL will be taken from the stock solution and transferred into 598 μL of diluent. However, if the final volume required is lower than the DF, or if

the amount to be pipetted from the stock solution is too low, then more than one dilution might be needed. The latter can be achieved by using the following equation:

Final DF = $DF_1 \times DF_2 \times DF_3 \times DF_4$ etc

For example, to prepare a dilution of 1:1,500 in a final volume of 400 μL step dilutions is needed. Here, the dilution steps can start with 1:15 then 1:100, meaning $15 \times 100 = 1,500$. Using the above formula:

400 μL/stock volume = 15

By rearranging the equation:

Stock volume = 400 μL/15 = 26.6 μL

This means to prepare 1:15 dilution, it must be in a volume of at least 26.6 μL. For example, add 0.3 μL from the stock solution into 29.7 μL of diluent. Subsequently, transfer 26.6 μL from the 1:100 prepared dilution into 373.4 μL of diluent (400–26.6 μL) resulting in a final dilution of 1:1,500

Serial Dilution

This method is used to generate several dilutions, in which the diluted stock solution prepared in the first step is used to prepare the next dilutions. Here, more than one equation is required including:

1. **Transfer volume = final volume/(DF − 1)**
2. **Diluent volume = final volume − transferred volume**
3. **Total volume = diluent volume + transfer volume**

For example, to prepare six-point dilutions of 1:4 with 50 μL per tube, 50 μL of the diluents will be needed, as the minimum volume for each step (volume needed per tube) plus additional volume for estimated pipetting errors, for instance, 50 μL, resulting in a desired diluent volume of 100 μL. Then the transfer volume and the total volume must be calculated.

For the **transfer volume**:

100 μL/(4 − 1) = 33.3 μL

For the **total volume**:

100 μL + 33.3 μL = 133.3 μL

The preparation steps are illustrated in Fig. 2.2.

General Safety Rules for Clinical Laboratories

Laboratory workers can be exposed to variety of hazards, including biological, chemical, physical, fire, explosive, and electrical. Therefore, it is essential for all personnel working in research, teaching or clinical laboratories to learn and apply all safety precautions and rules to maintain a safe daily working environment.

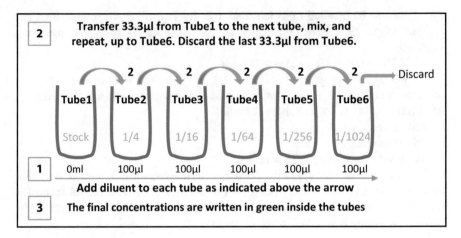

Fig. 2.2 Example of serial dilution

Upon handling samples, laboratory workers should follow the standard precautions, which may include:

1. Wearing gloves and changing them after handling samples that may contain high concentrations of microorganisms.
2. Before touching non-contaminated items and surfaces, and before leaving the laboratory, the gloves must be removed, followed by an immediate hand wash to prevent contamination.
3. A gown can protect skin and clothing, and must be removed if soiled followed by an immediate hand wash to avoid the spread of any microorganisms.
4. Procedures that may lead to blood sprays or splashes have to be performed with a mask, eye protection goggles, and a face shield to avoid the contact of any microorganisms with the mucous membrane of the eyes, nose, and mouth.
5. The hospital must have adequate procedures for routinely cleaning and disinfecting the surfaces (environmental control).
6. Sharp instruments or devices must be handled with care to prevent injuries. Therefore, never recap a needle, dispose syringes without removing the needle, do not bend or break needles, and dispose of all sharp items in puncture-resistant containers placed close to the area.

However, laboratory workers must be informed and well trained based on the type of hazards available in their workplace and according to their safety department's instructions and rules to avoid any possible injuries.

References

1. Novotny J, Handschumacher M, Bruccoleri RE. Protein antigenicity: a static surface property. Immunol Today. 1987;8(1):26–31.
2. Mahanty S, Prigent A, Garraud O. Immunogenicity of infectious pathogens and vaccine antigens. BMC Immunol. 2015;16:31.
3. Coico R, Sunshine G. Immunology: a short course. 7th ed. Chichester, West Sussex; Hoboken, NJ: John Wiley & Sons Inc.; 2015. p. 133.
4. Rossjohn J, Gras S, Miles JJ, Turner SJ, Godfrey DI, McCluskey J. T cell antigen receptor recognition of antigen-presenting molecules. Annu Rev Immunol. 2015;33:169–200.
5. Kambayashi T, Laufer TM. Atypical MHC class II-expressing antigen-presenting cells: can anything replace a dendritic cell? Nat Rev Immunol. 2014;14(11):719–30.
6. Chen H, He X, Wang Z, Wu D, Zhang H, Xu C, et al. Identification of human T cell receptor gammadelta-recognized epitopes/proteins via CDR3delta peptide-based immunobiochemical strategy. J Biol Chem. 2008;283(18):12528–37.
7. Schroeder HW Jr, Cavacini L. Structure and function of immunoglobulins. J Allergy Clin Immunol. 2010;125(2 Suppl 2):S41–52.

Study Questions

1. **Immunogens are:**

   (a) **Antigens.**
   (b) Not antigens.
   (c) Self-molecules.
   (d) None of the above.

2. **Foreign molecules are usually:**

   (a) **Immunogens.**
   (b) Tolerogen.
   (c) Hapten.
   (d) Carcinogen.

3. **For an antigen to be immunogenic:**

   (a) It has to be large and non-complex.
   (b) It has to be small and non-complex.
   (c) **It has to be large and complex.**
   (d) It has to resist enzymic degradation by APCs.

4. **Immunoglobulins are:**

   (a) Produced by the plasma cells.
   (b) Proteins.
   (c) Membranes bound or secreted.
   (d) **All the above.**

5. **The structure of an antibody consists of:**

   (a) **Two light chains and two heavy chains with Fab and Fc regions.**
   (b) One light chain and two heavy chains with the Fab and Fc regions.
   (c) Two light chains and one heavy chain with the Fab and Fc regions.
   (d) Two light chains and two heavy chains with the Fab region only.

6. **Interaction between a univalent antigen and its specific antibody can lead to:**

   (a) Precipitation.
   (b) Agglutination.
   (c) Complement activation.
   (d) **None of the above.**

7. **Antigen–antibody interaction is:**

   (a) Strong.
   (b) **Weak.**
   (c) Requires covalent bonding.
   (d) Does not involve electrostatic forces.

8. **Dilution in clinical laboratories can be prepared by using:**

   (a) The $C_1V_1 = C_2V_2$ method.
   (b) Serial dilution.
   (c) The dilution factor method.
   (d) **Any of the above methods.**

Chapter 3
Precipitation and Agglutination Reactions

Learning Objectives
By the end of this chapter the reader should be able to:

1. Understand the principle of precipitation.
2. Describe the different types of precipitation.
3. List several examples of the application of each precipitation technique.
4. State the principle of agglutination.
5. Explain the different types of agglutination and list the different tests that apply their principles.
6. List the advantages and disadvantages associated with agglutination.
7. Differentiate between agglutination and precipitation.
8. Describe the principle and types of hemagglutination.
9. List different tests that use the hemagglutination principle.

Most of the serological testing requires the interaction between antibodies and antigens to form visible antibody–antigen complexes. Several methods in clinical serology can detect antigen–antibody reactions, including:

1. Precipitation.
2. Agglutination.
3. Hemagglutination and hemagglutination inhibition.
4. Viral neutralization.
5. Radio-immunoassays.
6. Enzyme immunoassay and enzyme-linked immunosorbent assays.
7. Immunofluorescence.
8. Immunoblotting.
9. Immunochromatography.

© Springer International Publishing AG, part of Springer Nature 2018
R. Y. Alhabbab, *Basic Serological Testing*, Techniques in Life Science and
Biomedicine for the Non-Expert, https://doi.org/10.1007/978-3-319-77694-1_3

Precipitation Technique

Principle

The precipitation technique requires the formation of a visible lattice that results from the combination of soluble antigen to its soluble antibody [1–3]. It is usually works best when antigens and antibodies are at optimal proportions (**equivalence**) (Fig. 3.1) [2, 3].

The precipitation technique includes **ring precipitation** and **gel diffusion precipitation tests**.

Ring Precipitation Test

The ring precipitation test is usually performed in a tube, and requires the formation of antigen--antibody precipitate between two fluids as a ring of precipitate that is layered on the surface of the antibody (Fig. 3.2) [1, 2].

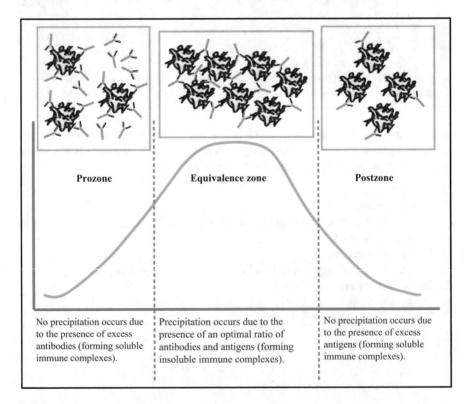

Prozone	Equivalence zone	Postzone
No precipitation occurs due to the presence of excess antibodies (forming soluble immune complexes).	Precipitation occurs due to the presence of an optimal ratio of antibodies and antigens (forming insoluble immune complexes).	No precipitation occurs due to the presence of excess antigens (forming soluble immune complexes).

Fig. 3.1 The influence of the ratio of antigen–antibodies on the formation of precipitation reaction

Fig. 3.2 The principle of
ring precipitation reaction

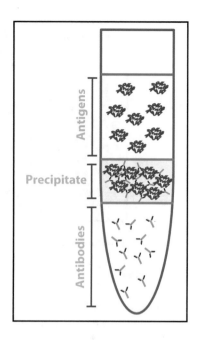

Application

A ring precipitation test is used for grouping streptococci and for determining
unknown proteins.

Gel Diffusion Precipitation Test

In gel diffusion precipitation tests, antibodies and antigens diffuse together in agar
medium forming a line of precipitate [2]. This test is available in two principles,
single diffusion and **double diffusion** [2].

Single Diffusion

In single diffusion, the antibodies are spread homogeneously in agar medium and
the antigens diffuse within the agar [2]. Here, the gel agar contains diluted antibodies specific to certain antigens [2]. A ring of precipitate forms upon the addition of
the antigens into the well, which is a cut in the agar [2]. The ring forms at the
equivalent point between the antibodies and the antigens [2]. The diameter of the
ring depends on the antigen concentration; thus, the higher antigen concentration,
the greater the diameter of the ring [2]. This test can provide the concentration of
antigens that is of interest in a patient's serum sample (Fig. 3.3).

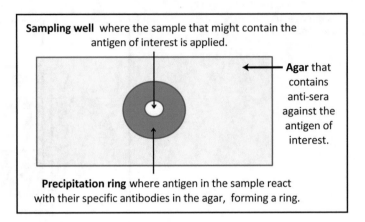

Fig. 3.3 Single-diffusion assays

Application

Single-diffusion assays, which are also called immunodiffusion assays, can be used to determine the concentration of immunoglobulins, complement components, and other serum proteins.

Double Diffusion

In double diffusion assays, antibodies and antigens are applied into two different wells in an agar medium and allowed to diffuse toward each other, forming a thin line of precipitate that meets at their equivalent point [2]. The concentration depends on the position of the line and the diffusion co-efficient of both the antibodies and the antigens (Fig. 3.4).

Application

This test is used to diagnose several fungal, viral and bacterial infections. In addition, it can be used to diagnose autoimmune diseases and to recognize *Corynebacterium diphtheriae*-produced toxins.

Agglutination

Principle

Agglutination is the development of antigen–antibody complexes in the form of particle clumps (agglutinates) due to the interaction between the insoluble form of antigens (i.e., antigen associated with latex particles) and its soluble and specific antibodies (Fig. 3.5) [1, 2].

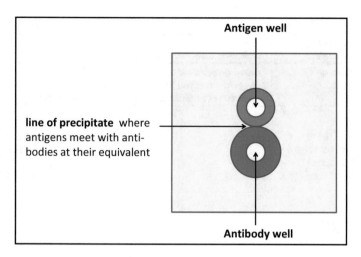

Fig. 3.4 Double-diffusion assay

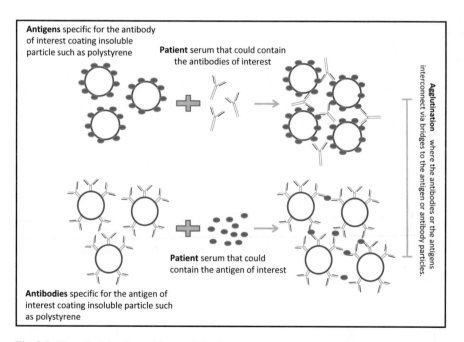

Fig. 3.5 The principle of a positive agglutination test

Agglutination is a semi-quantitative, sensitive, easy, and quick method. The agglutination reaction stage, which is also called the secondary phase, relies on the antigen's physical state, the concentration, the avidity of both antigens and antibodies, and the environment of the reaction (such as pH and protein concentration) [2]. The agglutination reaction can be direct or indirect.

Table 3.1 The advantages and limitations associated with the agglutination test

Advantages of agglutination test	Limitations associated with agglutination test
1. Easy and quick. 2. Sensitive.	1. Semi-quantitative test. 2. Agglutination can be inhibited owing to the presence of an extremely excessive number of antibodies (prozone).

Table 3.2 The major differences between agglutination and precipitation techniques

	Agglutination	Precipitation
Antigen	Insoluble	Soluble
Sensitivity	More sensitive	Less sensitive

Application

The agglutination test is used widely, for example, in detecting streptococci group B toxins, **rheumatoid arthritis**, and **C-reactive proteins**.

Direct Agglutination

In the **direct agglutination** test, the pathogen itself is used to detect specific antibodies against that pathogen [2]. The reaction between the patient-specific antibodies in the sera and the surface of the pathogen leads to the formation of visible clumps (agglutination) [2].

Indirect Agglutination

In the **indirect agglutination** technique, antigens or antibodies usually coat the surface of the latex or any other form of particles to detect the presence of specific antibodies or antigens of interest in the patient sera [2].

Table 3.1 illustrates the advantages and limitations of the agglutination test, whereas Table 3.2 shows the major differences between the agglutination and precipitation methods.

Hemagglutination

Principle

The **hemagglutination** test can be direct (viral hemagglutination) or indirect [1, 2, 4].

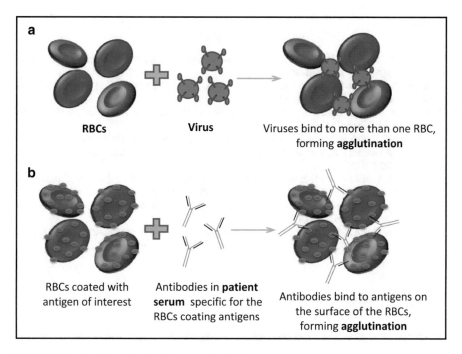

Fig. 3.6 The principle of the (**a**) direct and (**b**) indirect hemagglutination test

Direct Hemagglutination

Direct hemagglutination tests use the ability of some viruses to bind to red blood cells (RBCs), resulting in agglutination [1, 2]., such as the influenza virus, which can bind to fowl RBCs (Fig. 3.6a) [4].

Indirect Hemagglutination

Indirect hemagglutination requires the coating of the surface of the RBCs with the antigens of interest to detect their specific antibodies in patient serum (Fig. 3.6b) [1, 5, 6].

Application

Blood grouping, virus identification and in the detection of certain diseases.

References

1. Mak TW, Saunders ME. The immune response: basic and clinical principles. Amsterdam; Boston, MA: Elsevier/Academic; 2006. p. xx. 1194.
2. Coico R, Sunshine G. Immunology: a short course. 7th ed. Chichester, West Sussex; Hoboken, NJ: John Wiley & Sons Inc.; 2015.
3. Jacobsen C, Steensgaard J. Evidence of a two stage nature of precipitin reactions. Mol Immunol. 1979;16(8):571–6.
4. Klimov A, Balish A, Veguilla V, Sun H, Schiffer J. Lu X, et al. Influenza virus titration, antigenic characterization, and serological methods for antibody detection. Methods Mol Biol. 2012;865:25–51.
5. Mohan A, Saxena HM, Malhotra P. A comparison of titers of anti-Brucella antibodies of naturally infected and healthy vaccinated cattle by standard tube agglutination test, microtiter plate agglutination test, indirect hemagglutination assay, and indirect enzyme-linked immunosorbent assay. Vet World. 2016;9(7):717–22.
6. Singh DS, Das AK, Bhatia VN. Indirect haemagglutination test in the sero-diagnosis of amoebic and non-amoebic digestive disorders. J Assoc Physicians India. 1982;30(5):263–5.

Study Questions

1. **In the ring precipitation test, antigen interaction with antibodies occurs at:**

   (a) The top layer of the reaction tube.
   (b) **The middle layer of the reaction tube.**
   (c) The bottom layer of the reaction tube.
   (d) None of the above.

2. **Gel diffusion can be:**

   (a) Single.
   (b) Double.
   (c) Ring.
   (d) **a and b.**

3. **In the direct agglutination test:**

   (a) **Pathogen and patient antibodies form a clump.**
   (b) Latex coated particles detect the antibodies or the antigens in patient serum.
   (c) RBCs are used to form agglutination.
   (d) All the above.

4. **Indirect hemagglutination uses:**

   (a) Viruses as a binding agent.
   (b) **Coated RBCs with targeted antigens.**
   (c) Latex particles coated with targeted antigens.
   (d) Charcoal particles.

Chapter 4
Rapid Plasma Reagin (RPR) Test

Learning Objectives
By the end of this chapter the reader should be able to:

1. Identify RPR test applications, advantages, and limitations.
2. Describe RPR test principle.
3. List the reagents required for the RPR test.
4. List the general steps performed in the RPR test.
5. Differentiate between positive and negative RPR results.
6. Describe the major difference between the RPR and VDRL tests.

Syphilis is a sexually transmitted disease that also has the ability to pass from mother to fetus [1]. **Syphilis** is caused by bacteria called *Treponema pallidum* [2]. The infection has been reported to be asymptomatic in most patients [1]; therefore, serological testing is essential to screen for syphilis. Untreated syphilis infection can lead to severe complications in patients and pregnant mothers [1]. Syphilis can be detected using a **non-treponemal test** (non-specific screening test such as the **rapid plasma reagin, RPR,** test), or via a treponemal test (a specific test such as *Treponema pallidum* hemagglutination (TPHA)) test [3].

The RPR test is used in clinical laboratories as a quick, **screening, macroscopic**, non-treponemal test for syphilis [1, 4]. RPR is a non-treponemal test because it detects antibodies that are not specific to *T. pallidum*, but are released against phospholipid antigens such as a cardiolipin (cell membrane component), which is called reagin [1]. As anti-cardiolipins can be released in a variety of diseases associated with tissue damage, the RPR test is non-specific, non-treponemal test. Positive RPR or **Venereal Disease Research Laboratory (VDRL)** test results must be confirmed by a treponemal test such as TPHA, which uses specific *T. pallidum* antigens [1, 4].

© Springer International Publishing AG, part of Springer Nature 2018
R. Y. Alhabbab, *Basic Serological Testing*, Techniques in Life Science and
Biomedicine for the Non-Expert, https://doi.org/10.1007/978-3-319-77694-1_4

Rapid Plasma Reagin (RPR) Test

Principle

Rapid plasma reagin contains the same antigen suspension that is used by the VDRL test, another non-treponemal test used to screen for syphilis. VDRL antigen suspension contains cardiolipin [5]; however, in RPR the VDRL antigen suspension is modified with choline chloride to provide more stability [3, 4]. The cardiolipin is coated with charcoal particles to read the results without the need for a light microscope, unlike the results obtained from the VDRL test (Table 4.1) [3, 5]. The RPR test principle is explained in detail in Fig. 4.1.

RPR Test Reagents

1. Positive and negative controls.
2. Charcoal particles sensitized with cardiolipin.

Table 4.1 The major differences between the rapid plasma regain (RPR) and venereal disease research laboratory (VDRL) tests

	RPR	VDRL
Specimen	Serum/plasma	Serum/plasma
Sensitivity	More sensitive than VDRL	Less sensitive than RPR
Instruments required	A rotator	A light microscope

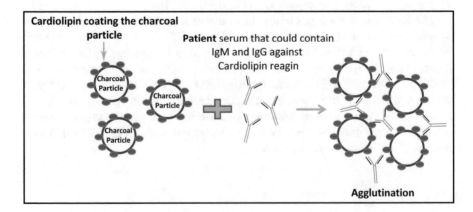

Fig. 4.1 Rapid plasma reagin test principle

Fig. 4.2 Rapid plasma
reagin test results

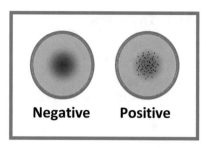

Negative   Positive

RPR Test Steps

1. Add the patient's serum, positive and negative controls independently to the appropriate circles of the test card.
2. Add one drop from the charcoal reagent to each circle and mix [4].
3. Incubate for 8 min on a rotator (100 rpm).
4. Read the results macroscopically (Fig. 4.2).

Note: these are the general steps followed in the RPR test, but always follow the quantities and instructions provided by the manufacturer.

The RPR and VDRL tests can give false-positive results. The most common conditions that may be associated with false-positive results include malaria, tuberculosis, viral fever, trypanosomiasis, leprosy, drug addiction, pregnancy, connective tissue diseases, and aging, and can all be a cause of cross-reactivity [1].

References

1. Herring A, Ballard R, Mabey D, Peeling RW, Initiative WTSTDD. Evaluation of rapid diagnostic tests: syphilis. Nat Rev Microbiol. 2006;4(12 Suppl):S33–40.
2. Peeling RW, Mabey DC. Syphilis. Nat Rev Microbiol. 2004;2(6):448–9.
3. Lee JH, Lim CS, Lee MG, Kim HS. Comparison of an automated rapid plasma reagin (RPR) test with the conventional RPR card test in syphilis testing. BMJ Open. 2014;4(12):e005664.
4. Larsen SA, Creighton ET. Rapid Plasma Reagin (RPR) 18-MM circle card test. CDC. 1996. Accessed 1 September 2017. Available from: https://www.cdc.gov/std/syphilis/manual-1998/chapt10.pdf.
5. Angue Y, Yauieb A, Mola G, Duke T, Amoa AB. Syphilis serology testing: a comparative study of Abbot Determine, Rapid Plasma Reagin (RPR) card test and Venereal Disease Research Laboratory (VDRL) methods. P N G Med J. 2005;48(3-4):168–73.

Study Questions

1. **Syphilis is transmitted:**

   (a) **Sexually.**
   (b) Via contaminated food.
   (c) Via droplet contact.
   (d) By the fecal–oral route.

2. **Syphilis is caused by:**

   (a) A virus called *Treponema pallidum*.
   (b) **Bacteria called *Treponema pallidum*.**
   (c) A fungus called *Treponema pallidum*.
   (d) A parasite called *Treponema pallidum*.

3. **The serological screening testing for syphilis is:**

   (a) **Rapid plasma reagin (RPR).**
   (b) *Treponema pallidum* hemagglutination (TPHA).
   (c) Enzyme-linked immunosorbent assay (ELISA).
   (d) Polymer chain reaction.

4. **RPR is a non-treponemal test because:**

   (a) RPR detects antibodies specific for *Treponema pallidum*.
   (b) **RPR detects antibodies against phospholipid antigens.**
   (c) RPR detects *Treponema pallidum* antigens directly.
   (d) None of the above.

5. **RPR and VDRL antigen suspension contains:**

   (a) **Cardiolipin.**
   (b) *Treponema pallidum*
   (c) Choline chloride.
   (d) Charcoal.

6. **RPR antigen suspension contains:**

   (a) Cardiolipin.
   (b) Choline chloride.
   (c) Charcoal.
   (d) **All the above.**

7. **VDRL results require:**

   (a) **A light microscope.**
   (b) Software for analysis.
   (c) An incubator.
   (d) A fridge.

Chapter 5
Treponema pallidum Hemagglutination (TPHA) Test

Learning Objectives
By the end of this chapter the reader should be able to:

1. Discuss the pathogenesis of syphilis.
2. Identify the *Treponema pallidum* hemagglutination (TPHA) test application.
3. Describe the TPHA test principle.
4. List the reagents required for the TPHA test.
5. List the general steps performed during the TPHA test.
6. Differentiate between positive and negative TPHA results.
7. Identify the TPHA test titer.

Syphilis is a sexually transmitted chronic infection that is caused by bacteria called *Treponema pallidum* [1]. Infection with *T. pallidum* progress through several stages. During the primary chancre, *T. pallidum* leads to an ulcer at the site of inoculation after an incubation of 21 days following exposure [1]. During this stage, anti-treponemal IgM and IgG antibodies can be detected 3 days following ulcer onset [2]. After approximately 6–8 weeks, the ulcer will resolve spontaneously (secondary stage) [1]. During the secondary stage, the infection spreads into any organ via the blood [1]. During this stage, IgG-specific antibodies increase disproportionately with a weak IgM antibody response [1]. Studies have confirmed that effective treatment at the primary and secondary stages during the infection is associated with decreasing to undetectable levels of IgM antibodies [3–5]. However, IgG antibodies can be circulating for years after treatment. Tertiary infection can occur several years later, affecting several tissues such as skin, bones or the central nervous and cardiovascular systems [1]. Positive rapid plasma reagin (RPR) or Venereal Disease Research Laboratory (VDRL) results must be confirmed using a **treponemal test** such as *Treponema pallidum* hemagglutination (**TPHA**), which uses specific *T. pallidum* antigens.

© Springer International Publishing AG, part of Springer Nature 2018
R. Y. Alhabbab, *Basic Serological Testing*, Techniques in Life Science and Biomedicine for the Non-Expert, https://doi.org/10.1007/978-3-319-77694-1_5

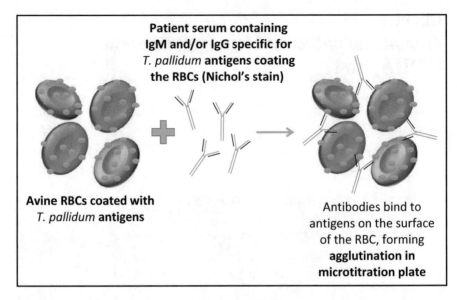

Patient serum containing IgM and/or IgG specific for *T. pallidum* antigens coating the RBCs (Nichol's stain)

Avine RBCs coated with *T. pallidum* antigens

Antibodies bind to antigens on the surface of the RBC, forming agglutination in microtitration plate

Fig. 5.1   The *Treponema pallidum* hemagglutination (TPHA) test principle

Treponema Pallidum **Hemagglutination (TPHA) Test**

Principle

A TPHA test is an indirect hemagglutination assay that uses *T. pallidum* sensitizing avian red blood cells (RBCs), which agglutinate with IgG and IgM antibodies in the patient's serum or plasma (Fig. 5.1) [6, 7]. TPHA can provide semi-quantitative or quantitative results.

Reagents That Must Be Provided in the Kit

1. TPHA test cells: avian RBCs coated with *T. pallidum* antigens [6, 7].
2. TPHA control cells: non-sensitized preserved avian RBCs used to detect a non-specific reaction [6, 7].
3. TPHA sample diluent.
4. TPHA positive and negative controls: human defibrinated plasma.

TPHA Test Steps

All the steps below may vary according to the manufacturer [6, 7].

1. Samples, controls, and reagents must reach room temperature before starting.
2. Put 100 µL of diluent in well 1 and 25 µL diluent in well 2 to well 10.
3. Add 25 µL of serum sample, positive and negative controls to well 1A, 1B, and 1C respectively. Mix and transfer 25 µL to well 2 to well 10 and discard the last 25 µL from well 10.
4. Add 75 µL of control cells to well 2.
5. Add 75 µL of test cells to well 3 to well 10.
6. Shake the plate and incubate for 45–60 min before reading the results.

Figure 5.2 illustrates the TPHA steps.

Results Interpretation

Positive results aggregate at the bottom of the well as a small mat (Fig. 5.3); the size of the mat indicates the strength of the positivity.

The cells for negative results are set at the bottom of the well (Fig. 5.3).

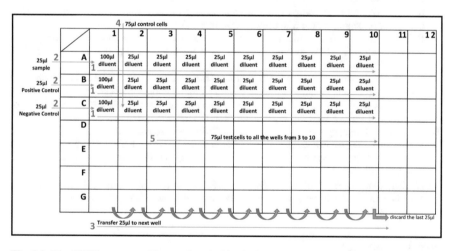

Fig. 5.2 The TPHA test steps. The numbers in *blue* indicate the sequence of the steps

Fig. 5.3 The TPHA test results

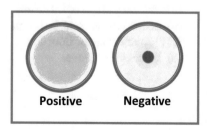

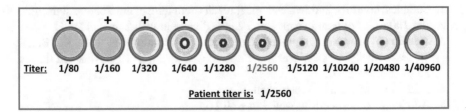

| Titer: | 1/80 | 1/160 | 1/320 | 1/640 | 1/1280 | 1/2560 | 1/5120 | 1/10240 | 1/20480 | 1/40960 |

Patient titer is: 1/2560

Fig. 5.4 The TPHA test results interpretation clarifying example

A non-specific reaction gives positive results with both control cells and test cells. A clarifying example is illustrated in Fig. 5.4.

References

1. Peeling RW, Mabey DC. Syphilis. Nat Rev Microbiol. 2004;2(6):448–9.
2. Sena AC, White BL, Sparling PF. Novel Treponema pallidum serologic tests: a paradigm shift in syphilis screening for the 21st century. Clin Infect Dis. 2010;51(6):700–8.
3. Baker-Zander SA, Roddy RE, Handsfield HH, Lukehart SA. IgG and IgM antibody reactivity to antigens of Treponema pallidum after treatment of syphilis. Sex Transm Dis. 1986;13(4):214–20.
4. Baughn RE, Jorizzo JL, Adams CB, Musher DM. Ig class and IgG subclass responses to Treponema pallidum in patients with syphilis. J Clin Immunol. 1988;8(2):128–39.
5. Merlin S, Andre J, Alacoque B, Paris-Hamelin A. Importance of specific IgM antibodies in 116 patients with various stages of syphilis. Genitourin Med. 1985;61(2):82–7.
6. BIOLABO. Haemagglutination assay for qualitative and semi-quantitative determination of antibodies to *Treponema pallidum* in human serum or plasma. BIOLABO. 2014. Accessed 2 September 2017. Available from: http://www.biolabo.fr/biolabo/pdfs/noticesE/syphilisE/AT-45-00-100-TPHA.
7. Human Diagnostics Worldwide. Syphilis TPHA liquid. Human-de. 2014. Accessed 2 September 2017. Available from: http://www.human-de.com/data/gb/vr/lx-tpha.pdf.

Study Questions

1. **Anti-treponemal IgM and IgG appears during:**

   (a) **Primary stage of infection.**
   (b) Secondary stage of infection.
   (c) Tertiary stage of infection.
   (d) None of the above.

2. *T. pallidum* **infection spreads through blood to any organs during:**

(a) The primary stage of infection.
(b) **The secondary stage of infection.**
(c) The tertiary stage of infection.
(d) All the above.

3. **Anti-treponemal IgG remains in the patient circulation:**

(a) **For several years after treatment.**
(b) For several days after treatment.
(c) During the infection only.
(d) For weeks after the infection.

4. *T. pallidum* **infection affects the body organs such as bones and skin during:**

(a) The primary stage of infection.
(b) The secondary stage of infection.
(c) **The tertiary stage of infection.**
(d) All the above.

5. **The TPHA test is performed:**

(a) For all patients suspected of having syphilis.
(b) **For patients with positive RPR or VDRL test results.**
(c) To confirm HIV infection.
(d) To test for *Brucella*.

6. **The TPHA test is:**

(a) **An indirect hemagglutination test.**
(b) A latex agglutination test.
(c) An ELISA-based assay.
(d) Molecular assay.

7. **The TPHA test uses:**

(a) **RBCs coated with *T. pallidum* antigens.**
(b) Latex particles coated with *T. pallidum* antigens.
(c) Charcoal particles coated with *T. pallidum* antigens.
(d) None of the above.

8. **Positive TPHA results:**

(a) Form clumps at the bottom of the well.
(b) Form latex agglutination on the reaction card.
(c) **Form a small mat at the bottom of the well.**
(d) Are set at the bottom of the well.

Chapter 6
Stained *Brucella* Suspensions

Learning Objectives
By the end of this chapter the reader should be able to:

1. Discuss the pathogenesis of brucellosis caused by the major pathogenic *Brucella* species to humans.
2. Describe the two main tests used for *Brucella* detection.
3. Describe the slide agglutination and SAT test principles.
4. List the reagents required for both slide agglutination and SAT tests.
5. List the general steps performed during both slide agglutination and SAT tests.
6. Differentiate between positive and negative slide agglutination and SAT test results.
7. Identify a SAT test titer.

Brucella is a facultative, intracellular, Gram-negative bacterium. The main four species that can lead to **zoonotic** brucellosis in several animal species and humans are *B. melitensis*, *B. suis*, *B. abortus*, and *B. canis* [1]. However, the most pathogenic species to humans are *B. melitensis*, *B. suis*, and *B. abortus*, while infection with *B. canis* is rare [2]. ***Brucella*** species are transmitted to humans via the consumption of unpasteurized contaminated milk, cheese, inhalation of infected aerosols, or via the contact with infected animals or their tissues [2]. Brucellosis is associated with common symptoms such as fever, asthenia, myalgia, arthralgia, sweats, lymphadenopathy, hepatomegaly, and splenomegaly [2]. In addition, brucellosis can cause osteoarticular manifestations that are common with the localized form of the disease, and in a few cases, can lead to neurobrucellosis, especially with *B. melitensis* [2–4]. Moreover, brucellosis can infect the liver in about 5–57% of the cases [5]. The main target cells for *Brucella* are macrophages and non-phagocytic epithelial cells [6]. *Brucella* is an intracellular bacterium that survives in their target cells, mainly via one of their virulent factors such as LPS (lipopolysaccharide) [7]. Cell-mediated immunity is the major protector against *Brucella* [7]. However,

© Springer International Publishing AG, part of Springer Nature 2018
R. Y. Alhabbab, *Basic Serological Testing*, Techniques in Life Science and
Biomedicine for the Non-Expert, https://doi.org/10.1007/978-3-319-77694-1_6

antibody-mediated immunity can provide partial protection, and can be used as a serological tool for the diagnoses of brucellosis [7].

Patients who have suspected brucellosis based on their clinical symptoms and their epidemiological link, or who had consumed contaminated dairy products, should undertake laboratory testing to confirm their cases [8].

The Most Pathogenic *Brucella* Species to Humans

Brucella abortus

The main host of *B. abortus* is cattle [1]. Therefore, infection can be transmitted to humans via any of the methods described above. In humans, symptoms of brucellosis caused by *B. abortus* can range from asymptomatic to a disease associated with flu-like symptoms [9]. Brucellosis caused by *B. abortus* is usually called **undulant fever** because of the unregulated/intermittent episodes of fever associated with the disease [9]. On the other hand, brucellosis caused by *B. abortus* in cattle leads to abortions and stillbirth [9].

Brucella melitensis

Brucella melitensis infects mainly sheep and goats, but they have the ability to infect a wide range of species in close contact such as cattle, camels, dogs, horses, and pigs [10]. Brucellosis caused by *B. melitensis* is called **Malta fever** or **Mediterranean fever** because it is very commonly spread in these areas [10]. In addition, it can be found in the Middle East and many other countries. *B. melitensis* can be transmitted to humans by contact or consumption of contaminated diary product [10].

In animals, *B. melitensis* can pass through placenta, leading to the birth of weak offspring, or result in abortion [10]. In humans, it can range from being asymptomatic to flu-like symptoms, or it could be associated with several complications such as arthritis and neurological signs [10]. In general, the symptoms are much more similar to those associated with *B. abortus*.

Brucella suis

Brucella suis mainly infects pigs [11]; infection with *B. abortus* or *B. melitensis* is rarely seen in pigs. Pigs with brucellosis suffer from abortion or stillbirth [11]. In humans, the symptoms are similar to those seen in *B. abortus* and *B. melitensis* infections [11].

Brucellosis Incubation Period

The incubation period for brucellosis is variable; however, it usually ranges from 2 weeks to 2 months or longer [12].

Serological Tests to Detect Brucellosis

The most commonly used and recommended tests by the CDC (Centers for Disease Control and Prevention) to confirm *Brucella* infection are:

1. **The serum agglutination test, tube (SAT),** or the modified version of the test, the *Brucella* microagglutination test.
2. **Slide agglutination test.**

Slide Agglutination Test

Principle

Antibodies specific to *Brucella* produced during brucellosis infection can be detected in a patient's serum through their agglutination with concentrated stained *Brucella* reagent (Fig. 6.1) [13].

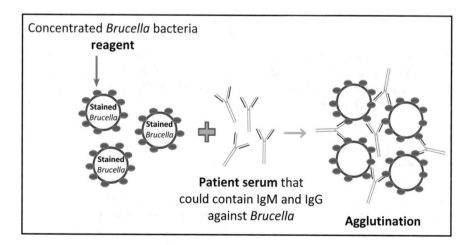

Fig. 6.1 Slide agglutination test principle

Reagents

The kit must provide:

1. Concentrated *Brucella* suspended in a buffered diluent and stained (depend on the manufacturer).
2. Positive control: diluted serum-containing antibodies to *Brucella* antigen (depending on the manufacturer).
3. Negative control: diluted serum non-reactive for *Brucella* antigens.
4. Six-well white slide.

Steps

The steps below may vary depending on the manufacturer's instructions [13].

1. Forty microliters of a patient's serum sample, positive and negative controls (may be provided as a dropper) to be placed on the appropriate circle of the six-well white slide.
2. After mixing the *Brucella* reagent, use the dropper provided and add one drop of the reagent to each sample, and for positive and negative controls.
3. Mix using a mixing stick.
4. Incubate for 4 min at room temperature on a rotator.
5. Look for agglutination under bright light.

Serum Agglutination Test, Tube (SAT)

The tube SAT is also called stained *Brucella* suspension. Tube SAT has an advantage over the slide agglutination test, which provides rapid, sensitive, and qualitative results. It is that tube SAT can detect the quantity of antibodies against *B. abortus* and *B. melitensis* in patient serum [14].

Principle

Serially diluted patient serum is mixed with bacterial suspension in a tube [14]. In the presence of sufficient antibodies, a visible agglutination occurs (Fig. 6.2).

Reagents

The kit must provide [14]:

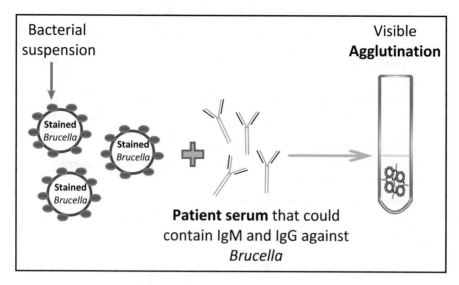

Fig. 6.2 Serum agglutination test principle

1. Stained *Brucella* suspensions, which consist of two-dropper bottles one for *B. abortus* and the second for *B. melitensis* (note: the suspension consists of killed stained bacteria).
2. Negative and positive controls (can be purchased separately).
3. Saline for dilution.

SAT Test Steps

1. Serially dilute the patient serum with the diluent provided in the kit or by using saline (Fig. 6.3), according to the manufacturer's instructions [14]. However, the general steps are the ones listed here.
2. Add one drop of *Brucella* suspension to each tube (tube 1 to tube 9).
3. After mixing, incubate in a water bath at 37 °C for 24 h.
4. Read the results.

   Note: tubes should not be stacked after incubation.

Results Interpretation

Positive samples and positive controls should provide granular agglutination. Negative samples and negative controls should show no change in the suspension appearance.

Positive controls should give agglutination and negative control suspension should be unchanged; otherwise, the test is invalid.

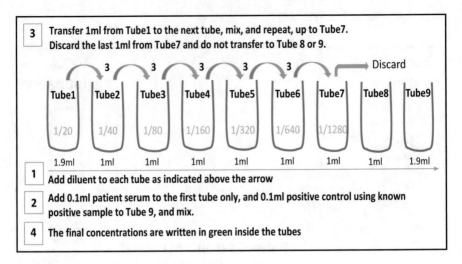

1	Add diluent to each tube as indicated above the arrow
2	Add 0.1ml patient serum to the first tube only, and 0.1ml positive control using known positive sample to Tube 9, and mix.
4	The final concentrations are written in green inside the tubes

Fig. 6.3 Serum agglutination test dilution steps

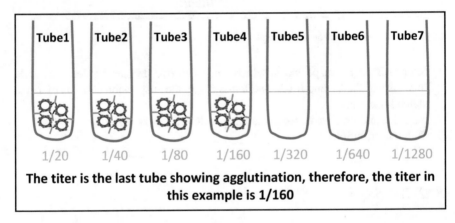

Tube1   Tube2   Tube3   Tube4   Tube5   Tube6   Tube7

1/20   1/40   1/80   1/160   1/320   1/640   1/1280

The titer is the last tube showing agglutination, therefore, the titer in this example is 1/160

Fig. 6.4 Serum agglutination test results interpretation example

Most healthy individuals are found to show agglutination; therefore, a titer less than 1/80 is considered insignificant [14].

Results Example

See Fig. 6.4 for the example of positive results interpretation.

References

1. He Y. Analyses of Brucella pathogenesis, host immunity, and vaccine targets using systems biology and bioinformatics. Front Cell Infect Microbiol. 2012;2:2.
2. Baldi PC, Giambartolomei GH. Pathogenesis and pathobiology of zoonotic brucellosis in humans. Rev Sci Tech. 2013;32(1):117–25.

3. Bouza E, Garcia de la Torre M, Parras F, Guerrero A, Rodriguez-Creixems M, Gobernado J. Brucellar meningitis. Rev Infect Dis. 1987;9(4):810–22.
4. Akhvlediani T, Clark DV, Chubabria G, Zenaishvili O, Hepburn MJ. The changing pattern of human brucellosis: clinical manifestations, epidemiology, and treatment outcomes over three decades in Georgia. BMC Infect Dis. 2010;10:346.
5. Akritidis N, Tzivras M, Delladetsima I, Stefanaki S, Moutsopoulos HM, Pappas G. The liver in brucellosis. Clin Gastroenterol Hepatol. 2007;5(9):1109–12.
6. Ko J, Splitter GA. Molecular host-pathogen interaction in brucellosis: current understanding and future approaches to vaccine development for mice and humans. Clin Microbiol Rev. 2003;16(1):65–78.
7. Lapaque N, Moriyon I, Moreno E, Gorvel JP. Brucella lipopolysaccharide acts as a virulence factor. Curr Opin Microbiol. 2005;8(1):60–6.
8. Fiori PL, Mastrandrea S, Rappelli P, Cappuccinelli P. Brucella abortus infection acquired in microbiology laboratories. J Clin Microbiol. 2000;38(5):2005–6.
9. The Center for Food Security and Public Health. Bovine brucellosis: *Brucella abortus*. CFSPH. 2009. Accessed 4 September 2017. Available from: http://www.cfsph.iastate.edu/Factsheets/pdfs/brucellosis_abortus.pdf.
10. The Center for Food Security and Public Health. Ovine and caprine brucellosis: *Brucella melitensis*. CFSPH. 2009. Accessed 4 September 2017. Available from: http://www.cfsph.iastate.edu/Factsheets/pdfs/brucellosis_melitensis.pdf.
11. The Center for Food Security and Public Health. Porcine and rangiferine brucellosis: *Brucella suis*. CFSPH. 2009. Accessed 4 September 2017. Available from: http://www.cfsph.iastate.edu/Factsheets/pdfs/brucellosis_suis.pdf.
12. World Health Organization (WHO). Brucellosis (human). WHO. 2005. Accessed 4 September 2017. Available from: http://www.who.int/zoonoses/diseases/Brucellosissurveillance.pdf.
13. Vircell microbiologists. Rose Bengal. 2005. Accessed 4 September 2017. Available from: http://www.peramed.com/peramed/docs/RB001_8436040325766_EN.pdf.
14. Thermo Fisher Scientific. Stained Brucella suspensions. Thermo Fisher. 2013. Accessed 4 September 2017. Available from: https://tools.thermofisher.com/content/sfs/manuals/X7817.pdf.

Study Questions

1. *Brucella* is:

   (a) An intracellular Gram-positive bacterium.
   (b) **An intracellular Gram-negative bacterium.**
   (c) An extracellular Gram-positive bacterium.
   (d) An intracellular virus.

2. *Brucella* is transmitted via:

   (a) Sexual contact.
   (b) Fecal–oral route.
   (c) **Consumption of contaminated milk.**
   (d) None of the above.

3. **The main target cells for *Brucella* are:**

   (a) B cells.
   (b) T cells.
   (c) Neutrophils.
   (d) **Macrophages.**

4. *Brucella* virulent factor is:

   (a) **LPS.**
   (b) Cytolysin.
   (c) Protease.
   (d) Exotoxin.

5. **The major protector against *Brucella* is:**

   (a) **Cell-mediated immunity.**
   (b) Humoral-mediated immunity.
   (c) Passive immunity.
   (d) None of the above.

6. **Brucellosis caused by *B. abortus* is called:**

   (a) **Undulant fever.**
   (b) Malta fever.
   (c) Mediterranean.
   (d) Yellow fever.

7. **Brucellosis caused by *B. melitensis* is called:**

   (a) Undulant fever.
   (b) **Malta fever.**
   (c) Yellow fever.
   (d) None of the above.

8. **The slide agglutination test used to detect *Brucella* is:**

   (a) Latex agglutination.
   (b) **Bacteria particle agglutination.**
   (c) ELISA-based.
   (d) Hemagglutination.

9. **Serum agglutination test (SAT) that detects *Brucella* is:**

   (a) **Quantitative.**
   (b) Qualitative.
   (c) Non-specific.
   (d) All the above.

10. **SAT results less than 1/80 titer are considered:**

    (a) **Non-significant.**
    (b) Significant.
    (c) Specific.
    (d) None of the above.

Chapter 7
Rheumatoid Factor (RF)

Learning Objectives
By the end of this chapter the reader should be able to:

1. Discuss the pathogenesis of rheumatoid arthritis.
2. Describe the rheumatoid factor (RF) latex agglutination test principle.
3. List the reagents required for the RF latex agglutination test.
4. List the general steps performed during the RF latex agglutination test.
5. Differentiate between positive and negative RF latex agglutination test results.

Autoimmune disorders occur because of the inability of the immune system to discriminate between self-antigens and non-self-antigens. Therefore, the immune system starts to attack self-antigens such as joints. **Rheumatoid arthritis (RA)** is one of the most widely spread chronic autoimmune disorders [1]. In RA, the synovium, the thin membrane, is a few cells thick and surrounds the joints and the tendon sheaths, undergoes **chronic inflammation** owing to the chronic infiltration of the inflammatory cells to the area [1]. The key player cells involved in RA are T cells, in particular Th17, macrophages, and B cells [1]. B cells produce specific autoantibodies, which play a critical role in the pathogenesis of the disease [2]. For example, the **rheumatoid factor (RF)** consists of **autoantibodies** that are produced by the B cells during RA and can interact with the Fc region of the self-IgG antibodies [2]. Therefore, RF has been used as a biomarker for RA. Recently, an additional autoantibody has been identified to be associated with RA, called **anti-citrullinated protein antibody (ACPA)**, but it is not as common as RF in clinical laboratories [3–7].

Currently, the most common test used in clinical laboratories to detect RF is latex agglutination [8]. However, the latex agglutination test does not provide high sensitivity and does not differentiate between the various classes of RF (IgA, IgG or IgM), which can be detected by ELISA [8]. Nevertheless, in this chapter, the **RF latex agglutination test** is discussed and ELISA is explained elsewhere.

© Springer International Publishing AG, part of Springer Nature 2018
R. Y. Alhabbab, *Basic Serological Testing*, Techniques in Life Science and
Biomedicine for the Non-Expert, https://doi.org/10.1007/978-3-319-77694-1_7

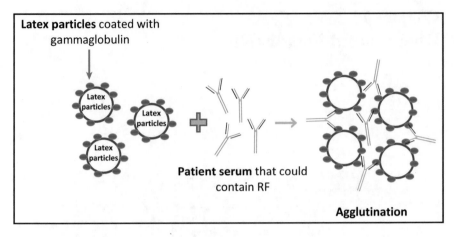

Fig. 7.1   The principle of the rheumatoid factor latex agglutination test

RF Latex Agglutination Test

Principle

The RF latex agglutination test is a qualitative and semi-quantitative test for detecting RF. Here, human gamma globulin coats latex particles. The mixing of these latex particles with patient serum that contains RF results in visual agglutination (Fig. 7.1).

The Application of the RF Latex Agglutination Test

The RF latex agglutination test is used to detect RA in patients. However, RF can also be detected in other diseases, and in healthy people. Therefore, it is always recommended to measure other antibodies together with RF to improve the diagnostic accuracy. Nevertheless, RF can be used to monitor RA patients after being diagnosed, to aid in their therapy [9].

Reagents and Materials Used

1. Latex reagent: latex particles coated with human gamma globulin.
2. Positive control: serum-containing RF.
3. Negative control: animal serum.
4. Slide test.

Fig. 7.2 Positive and negative results of the rheumatoid factor latex agglutination test

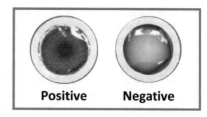

RF Latex Agglutination Test Steps

1. All reagents, samples, and controls must reach room temperature.
2. Add one drop or 20–50 µl (depending on the manufacturer's instructions) to the appropriate circles on the test slide.
3. Mix the latex reagent gently before using and add one drop or as specified by the manufacturer to each sample to be tested.
4. Mix the drops.
5. Incubate the slide test for 2 min on a rotator at room temperature.
6. Read the results.

Results Interpretation

Patient serum containing RF and positive controls should develop agglutination with the latex particles.

On the other hand, negative control and serum with no RF do not form agglutination with latex particles (Fig. 7.2).

RF Latex Agglutination Test Limitations

1. Not all serum obtained from a patient with RA contains RF.
2. RF can be detected with other diseases and infections such as **mononucleosis**.

References

1. Isaacs JD. The changing face of rheumatoid arthritis: sustained remission for all? Nat Rev Immunol. 2010;10(8):605–11.
2. Burska AN, Hunt L, Boissinot M, Strollo R, Ryan BJ, Vital E, et al. Autoantibodies to post-translational modifications in rheumatoid arthritis. Mediat Inflamm. 2014;2014:492873.
3. Nissim A, Winyard PG, Corrigall V, Fatah R, Perrett D, Panayi G, et al. Generation of neoanti-genic epitopes after posttranslational modification of type II collagen by factors present within the inflamed joint. Arthritis Rheum. 2005;52(12):3829–38.

4. Marcinkiewicz J, Biedron R, Maresz K, Kwasny-Krochin B, Bobek M, Kontny E, et al. Oxidative modification of type II collagen differentially affects its arthritogenic and tolerogenic capacity in experimental arthritis. Arch Immunol Ther Exp. 2004;52(4):284–91.
5. Anderton SM. Post-translational modifications of self antigens: implications for autoimmunity. Curr Opin Immunol. 2004;16(6):753–8.
6. Shi J, Knevel R, Suwannalai P, van der Linden MP, Janssen GM, van Veelen PA, et al. Autoantibodies recognizing carbamylated proteins are present in sera of patients with rheumatoid arthritis and predict joint damage. Proc Natl Acad Sci U S A. 2011;108(42):17372–7.
7. Eggleton P, Nissim A, Ryan BJ, Whiteman M, Winyard PG. Detection and isolation of human serum autoantibodies that recognize oxidatively modified autoantigens. Free Radic Biol Med. 2013;57:79–91.
8. Abnova. Rheumatoid Factoer IgG ELISA kit. Available from: http://www.abnova.com/protocol_pdf/KA1288.pdf. Accessed 6 Sept 2017.
9. Ingegnoli F, Castelli R, Gualtierotti R. Rheumatoid factors: clinical applications. Dis Markers. 2013;35(6):727–34.

Study Questions

1. **Rheumatoid arthritis is:**

   (a) Acute autoimmune disease.
   (b) **Chronic autoimmune disease.**
   (c) Chronic allergic disease.
   (d) Viral infection.

2. **The key player cells involved in rheumatoid arthritis pathogenesis are:**

   (a) Th17 cells.
   (b) B cells.
   (c) Macrophages.
   (d) **All the above.**

3. **Rheumatoid factor is:**

   (a) An enzyme produced in rheumatoid arthritis.
   (b) A cytokine produced in rheumatoid arthritis.
   (c) **An Autoantibody produced in rheumatoid arthritis.**
   (d) None of the above.

4. **Rheumatoid factor is an autoantibody against:**

   (a) DNA.
   (b) Lipids in the cell membrane.
   (c) Red blood cells.
   (d) **Fc region of IgG antibodies.**

5. **Rheumatoid factor is detected in clinical laboratories by:**

   (a) PCR.
   (b) **The latex agglutination test.**

(c) Hemagglutination.
(d) Radial immunodiffusion.

6. **In the rheumatoid factor latex agglutination test, the latex particles are coated with:**

   (a) **Gamma globulin.**
   (b) Toxin.
   (c) Bacterial antigen.
   (d) All the above.

7. **All the following statements about the rheumatoid factor latex agglutination test are false, except:**

   (a) Rheumatoid factor can be detected only in rheumatoid arthritis patients.
   (b) Rheumatoid factor can be detected in all rheumatoid arthritis patients.
   (c) **Rheumatoid factor is used to monitor rheumatoid arthritis patients.**
   (d) All the above.

Chapter 8
Suspension Anti-Streptolysin-O (ASO/ASL) Test

Learning Objectives
By the end of this chapter the reader should be able to:

1. Discuss the pathogenesis of group A streptococcus (GAS).
2. Describe the ASO/ASL test principle.
3. List the reagents required for the ASO/ASL test.
4. List the general steps performed during the ASO/ASL test.
5. Differentiate between positive and negative ASO/ASL test results.

Group A streptococcus (GAS) is a Gram-positive bacterium that is also known as *Streptococcus pyogenes* [1]. Several diseases with various clinical manifestations can be caused by GAS, such as acute **glomerulonephritis** and **rheumatic fever** [1–3]. GAS infection can range from mild pharyngitis and impetigo to severe post-streptococcal sequelae [4]. The host immune system response to GAS infection is complex and relies mainly on neutrophils, macrophages, and dendritic cells [5–8]. The activation and role of these cells depend mainly on their pattern recognition receptors (PRRs) interaction with pathogen-associated molecular patterns (PAMPs) derived from GAS [4]. The pathogenesis of GAS depends on the production of cell surface virulence factors and on the secretion of several virulence factors [9]. Molecules that are produced by GAS and facilitate their adhesion to the host cells and molecules that can interfere with host immunity are considered cell-surface virulence factors, whereas secreted virulence factors include **super-antigens** such as **streptolysin O (SLO)** [9]. SLO is a cytolysin that binds to cholesterol located in the host plasma membrane resulting in the formation of large pores that eventually lead to cell apoptosis [9].

Additionally, SLO helps GAS to escape from the **endosome-lysosome mechanism** of killing in host cells after invading them [10–13]. Several adaptive immune responses are associated with GAS such as the production of antibodies specific to SLO by B cells [14]. Therefore, **anti-streptolysin O (ASO/ASL)** is the most commonly used antibody in clinical laboratories for identifying the existence of GAS infection and for confirming previous exposure [3].

© Springer International Publishing AG, part of Springer Nature 2018
R. Y. Alhabbab, *Basic Serological Testing*, Techniques in Life Science and
Biomedicine for the Non-Expert, https://doi.org/10.1007/978-3-319-77694-1_8

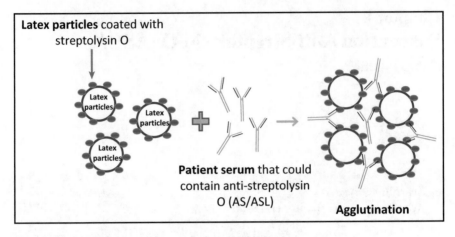

Fig. 8.1 The principle of the antistreptolysin O (ASO/ASL) test

ASO/ASL Test

Principle

The ASO/ASL test uses polystyrene latex particles coated with streptolysin O that develop agglutination upon interacting with ASO/ASL in patient serum (Fig. 8.1) [15, 16]. The ASO/ASL test provides qualitative and semi-quantitative results [15, 16].

ASO/ASL Test Application

1. The ASO/ASL test is the best for determining antecedent GAS infection [3].
2. The ASO titer is high in 80–95% of patients with acute rheumatic fever and acute glomerulonephritis [3].

ASO/ASL Test Reagents

1. Latex reagent: latex particles coated with SLO.
2. Positive and negative controls.
3. Test slide.

ASO/ASL Test Steps

1. All reagents, samples, and controls must reach room temperature.

2. Place one drop of each control and 10–50 µl of patient serum into the appropriate labeled circle on the test slide.
3. Add one drop of latex reagent (after mixing by inverting the bottle several times) to each circle, including controls and samples.
4. After mixing, incubate the slide test for 2–5 min at room temperature on a rotator.
5. Read the results.

Results Interpretation

The presence of agglutination indicates that the serum contains ASO (Fig. 7.2). Positive samples are required to be re-tested in semi-quantitative tests, which use the same principle and steps as above with only one difference: that the patient serum should be serially diluted.

References

1. Cole JN, Barnett TC, Nizet V, Walker MJ. Molecular insight into invasive group A streptococcal disease. Nat Rev Microbiol. 2011;9(10):724–36.
2. Carapetis JR, Steer AC, Mulholland EK, Weber M. The global burden of group A streptococcal diseases. Lancet Infect Dis. 2005;5(11):685–94.
3. Cunningham MW. Pathogenesis of group A streptococcal infections. Clin Microbiol Rev. 2000;13(3):470–511.
4. Fieber C, Kovarik P. Responses of innate immune cells to group A Streptococcus. Front Cell Infect Microbiol. 2014;4:140.
5. Goldmann O, Rohde M, Chhatwal GS, Medina E. Role of macrophages in host resistance to group A streptococci. Infect Immun. 2004;72(5):2956–63.
6. Loof TG, Rohde M, Chhatwal GS, Jung S, Medina E. The contribution of dendritic cells to host defenses against Streptococcus pyogenes. J Infect Dis. 2007;196(12):1794–803.
7. Zinkernagel AS, Timmer AM, Pence MA, Locke JB, Buchanan JT, Turner CE, et al. The IL-8 protease SpyCEP/ScpC of group A Streptococcus promotes resistance to neutrophil killing. Cell Host Microbe. 2008;4(2):170–8.
8. Mishalian I, Ordan M, Peled A, Maly A, Eichenbaum MB, Ravins M, et al. Recruited macrophages control dissemination of group A Streptococcus from infected soft tissues. J Immunol. 2011;187(11):6022–31.
9. Brosnahan AJ, Schlievert PM. Gram-positive bacterial superantigen outside-in signaling causes toxic shock syndrome. FEBS J. 2011;278(23):4649–67.
10. Bhakdi S, Tranum-Jensen J, Sziegoleit A. Mechanism of membrane damage by streptolysin-O. Infect Immun. 1985;47(1):52–60.
11. Timmer AM, Timmer JC, Pence MA, Hsu LC, Ghochani M, Frey TG, et al. Streptolysin O promotes group A Streptococcus immune evasion by accelerated macrophage apoptosis. J Biol Chem. 2009;284(2):862–71.
12. Hakansson A, Bentley CC, Shakhnovic EA, Wessels MR. Cytolysin-dependent evasion of lysosomal killing. Proc Natl Acad Sci U S A. 2005;102(14):5192–7.

13. Nakagawa I, Amano A, Mizushima N, Yamamoto A, Yamaguchi H, Kamimoto T, et al. Autophagy defends cells against invading group A Streptococcus. Science. 2004;306(5698):1037–40.
14. Zafindraibe NJ, Randriamanantany ZA, Rajaonatahina DH, Andriamahenina R, Rasamindrakotroka A. Current practice about the evaluation of antibody to streptolysin O (ASO) levels by physicians working in Antananarivo, Madagascar. Afr Health Sci. 2014;14(2):384–9.
15. Spectrum. Antistreptolysin O Titre (ASOT), s rspid lstex slide test for the detection of anti-streptolysin O antibodies in serum. Spectrum-diagnostics. 2011. Available from: http://spectrum-diagnostics.com/data/ASOT.pdf. Accessed 7 September 2017
16. Archem diagnostic. Antistreptolysin O (ASO). falezmedkal. 2010. Available from: http://www.falezmedikal.com/pdflerLab/5345880389.pdf. Accessed 7 September 2017

Study Questions

1. **Group A streptococcal secreted virulence factor includes:**

    (a) **Superantigens such as streptolysin O**.
    (b) Lysosome.
    (c) DNAase.
    (d) Proteinase.

2. **Streptolysin O leads to:**

    (a) **Cell apoptosis**.
    (b) Cell proliferation.
    (c) DNA degradation.
    (d) None of the above.

3. **The most commonly used serological marker in the ASO/ASL test is:**

    (a) Anti-streptococcus.
    (b) **Anti-streptolysin O**.
    (c) Anti-GAS (group A streptococcus).
    (d) All the above.

4. **ASO/ASL test is:**

    (a) **Latex agglutination test**.
    (b) Hemagglutination assay.
    (c) Molecular assay.
    (d) Immunodiffusion test.

5. **ASO/ASL reagent consist of:**

    (a) **Polystyrene latex particles coated with SLO**.
    (b) Charcoal particles coated with SLO.
    (c) Red blood cells coated with SLO.
    (d) None of the above.

Chapter 9
C-Reactive Protein (CRP) Latex Agglutination Test

Learning Objectives
By the end of this chapter the reader should be able to:

1. Discuss the process of CRP production.
2. Describe the principle of the CRP latex agglutination test.
3. List the reagents required for the CRP latex agglutination test.
4. List the general steps performed during the CRP latex agglutination test.
5. Differentiate between positive and negative CRP latex agglutination test results.

During inflammation, the immune cells, mainly the innate cells, produce several cytokines such as IL-6, IL-1 and TNF-α, which in turn activate the liver cells to produce **acute phase proteins** including **C-reactive proteins (CRPs)** [1, 2]. Therefore, CRPs are not directly associated with a specific disease. In clinical laboratories, CRPs are used as a marker for inflammation. However, several chronic diseases have been associated with an elevated level of CRPs, such as cancer [3, 4]. Currently, clinical laboratories are using an assay with high sensitivity in detecting even very low levels of CRP called **hsCRP** [5]. Several studies have recommended the use of hsCRP in cardiovascular disease (CVD) risk prediction because inflammation plays an important role in the initiation and progression of CVD and atherothrombosis [5–9]. CRP can be detected by the latex agglutination test or ELISA. However, the most commonly used test in clinical laboratories is latex agglutination.

© Springer International Publishing AG, part of Springer Nature 2018   59
R. Y. Alhabbab, *Basic Serological Testing*, Techniques in Life Science and
Biomedicine for the Non-Expert, https://doi.org/10.1007/978-3-319-77694-1_9

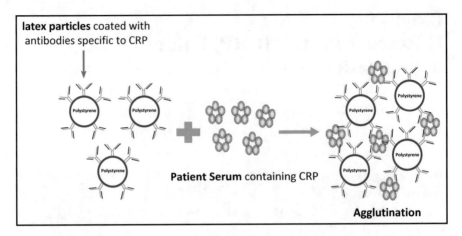

Fig. 9.1 The principle of the CRP latex agglutination test

CRP Latex Agglutination Test

Principle

The CRP latex agglutination assay is a qualitative and semi-quantitative test. The latex particles used in the CRP latex agglutination test are coated with anti-human CRP that agglutinate upon mixing with patient serum containing CRP (Fig. 9.1) [10].

Applications and Significance

The detection of CRP level by a latex agglutination test is mostly used as marker for active inflammation.

Reagents

1. Latex reagent: latex particles coated with anti-human CRP.
2. Positive and negative controls.
3. Test slide.

Test Steps

1. Bring all reagents, controls, and samples to room temperature.

2. Place one drop of the positive and the negative controls and 20–50 µl (depending on the manufacturer's instructions) from the patient serum into the appropriate circle on the test slide.
3. Swirl the latex reagent.
4. Add one drop from the latex reagent to each circle.
5. Mix and incubate for 2–5 min on a rotator at room temperature.
6. Read the results.

Results Interpretation

The presence of agglutination indicates a CRP concentration of 6 mg/l (may be higher or lower depending on the manufacturer's instructions).

References

1. Guo L, Liu S, Zhang S, Chen Q, Zhang M, Quan P, et al. C-reactive protein and risk of breast cancer: a systematic review and meta-analysis. Sci Rep. 2015;5:10508.
2. Mahmoud FA, Rivera NI. The role of C-reactive protein as a prognostic indicator in advanced cancer. Curr Oncol Rep. 2002;4(3):250–5.
3. Heikkila K, Harris R, Lowe G, Rumley A, Yarnell J, Gallacher J, et al. Associations of circulating C-reactive protein and interleukin-6 with cancer risk: findings from two prospective cohorts and a meta-analysis. Cancer Causes Control. 2009;20(1):15–26.
4. Poole EM, Lee IM, Ridker PM, Buring JE, Hankinson SE, Tworoger SS. A prospective study of circulating C-reactive protein, interleukin-6, and tumor necrosis factor alpha receptor 2 levels and risk of ovarian cancer. Am J Epidemiol. 2013;178(8):1256–64.
5. Yousuf O, Mohanty BD, Martin SS, Joshi PH, Blaha MJ, Nasir K, et al. High-sensitivity C-reactive protein and cardiovascular disease: a resolute belief or an elusive link? J Am Coll Cardiol. 2013;62(5):397–408.
6. Pepys MB, Hirschfield GM. C-reactive protein: a critical update. J Clin Invest. 2003;111(12):1805–12.
7. Kuller LH, Tracy RP, Shaten J, Meilahn EN. Relation of C-reactive protein and coronary heart disease in the MRFIT nested case-control study. Multiple Risk Factor Intervention Trial. Am J Epidemiol. 1996;144(6):537–47.
8. Musunuru K, Kral BG, Blumenthal RS, Fuster V, Campbell CY, Gluckman TJ, et al. The use of high-sensitivity assays for C-reactive protein in clinical practice. Nat Clin Pract Cardiovasc Med. 2008;5(10):621–35.
9. Ridker PM, Cushman M, Stampfer MJ, Tracy RP, Hennekens CH. Inflammation, aspirin, and the risk of cardiovascular disease in apparently healthy men. N Engl J Med. 1997;336(14):973–9.
10. Pulse scientific INC. C-Reactive Protein (CRP) Latex Test. Pulsescientific. Available from: file:///Users/drr/Downloads/Pulse_Latex_CRP_Instructions_en.pdf. Accessed 11 September 2017.

Study Questions

1. **During inflammation, the liver cells are activated by:**

   (a) T and B cell.
   (b) **IL-6 and IL-1**.
   (c) IL-10 and TGF-β.
   (d) Complements.

2. **All the following statements about CRP are true, except:**

   (a) CRP is produced by the liver cells.
   (b) CRP is an acute phase protein.
   (c) **CRP is associated with specific diseases**.
   (d) CRP is produced during inflammation.

3. **hsCRP can be used:**

   (a) As an inflammation marker.
   (b) To assess cardiovascular disease risk.
   (c) To detect atherothrombosis.
   (d) **All the above**.

4. **CRP is detected by:**

   (a) **The latex agglutination test**.
   (b) The hemagglutination test.
   (c) A molecular assay.
   (d) An immunofluorescent assay.

5. **The reagent used in the CRP latex agglutination test consists of:**

   (a) Latex particles coated with CRP.
   (b) **Latex particles coated with anti-CRP**.
   (c) Latex particles coated with inflammatory cytokines.
   (d) None of the above.

Chapter 10
Complement Fixation Test (CFT)

Learning Objectives
By the end of this chapter the reader should be able to:

1. Describe the principle of the complement fixation test (CFT).
2. List the reagents required for CFT.
3. List the general steps performed during CFT.
4. Differentiate between positive and negative CFT results.

Complement fixation assays are used to measure the level of specific antibodies that have been produced in response to certain infections such as viral infections.

Complement Fixation Test

Principle

Patient serum usually contains complements; therefore, the patient samples should be pre-heated to destroy all the complements without affecting the antibodies and the antigens in the serum. Subsequently, pre-heated serum is mixed with standard antigens and complements. Patient antibodies opsonize the standard antigens, and complements become fixed on the surface of the opsonizing antibodies. Complement remains unfixed when antibodies are absent from patient serum [1].

Sheep red blood cells (sRBCs) sensitized with specific antibodies to sRBCs are used as an indicator system to detect any residual of the unfixed complement remaining in the reaction [1]. Therefore, unfixed complements bind to sensitized sRBCs and lyse them, while the presence of antibodies in patient serum consumes the available complement in the reaction, resulting in visually intact sRBCs (Fig. 10.1) [1].

© Springer International Publishing AG, part of Springer Nature 2018
R. Y. Alhabbab, *Basic Serological Testing*, Techniques in Life Science and
Biomedicine for the Non-Expert, https://doi.org/10.1007/978-3-319-77694-1_10

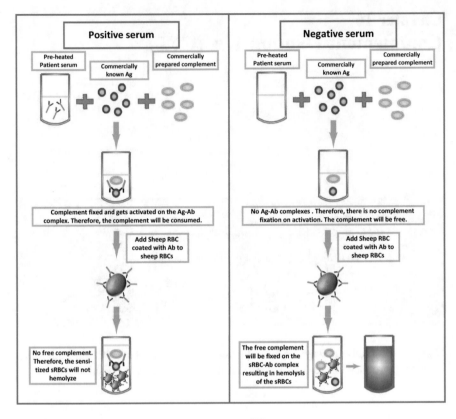

Fig. 10.1 Principle of the complement fixation test (CFT)

Reagents Provided in the Kit

1. Complements, usually from guinea pigs.
2. Sheep RBCs.
3. Sensitized sheep RBCs.
4. Standard antigens.
5. CFT control antisera.
6. Buffer.

Preparation of CFT Reagents

The procedure may vary between manufacturers. To obtain optimal results, reagents such as complement, sensitized sRBCs, sRBCs, and standard antigens must be standardized.

Preparation of Complement and Sensitized sRBCs [1]

1. Two-dimensional titration is usually used to determine the optimal concentration of complement and sensitized sRBCs. Complement is usually provided in lyophilized form; therefore, it has to be re-constituted with distilled water (dH_2O) (as per the manufacturer's instructions). To obtain an accurate end-point the complement dilutions are prepared at 20% differences in concentration, as illustrated in Fig. 10.2.
2. Setting up titration of complement and sensitized sRBCs. For complement preparation, use a microtiter plate to perform this step, as shown in Fig. 10.3. After mixing the microtiter plate contents as indicated in Fig. 10.3, incubate the plate overnight at 4 °C. During the incubation, prepare the sensitized sRBCs, first by diluting sRBC-specific antibodies (**hemolysin**) in tubes, as shown in Fig. 10.4. After preparing 4% sRBCs (4 ml sRBCs plus 8 ml buffer), sensitize them with hemolysin in tubes (bijou tubes), as shown in Fig. 10.5.
3. After overnight incubation, place the plate at 37 °C for 30 min, then gently re-suspend the prepared sensitized sRBCs.
4. After a 30-min incubation, add 25 µl from the sensitized sRBCs into the microtiter plate, as illustrated in Fig. 10.6.
5. Mix and incubate 30 min at 37 °C. Re-apply mixing at 10, 20, and at the end of the incubation time.
6. Centrifuge to settle the cells.
7. Read the degree of hemolysis by scoring as following:

0 = total lysis 100%.
Trace = 99–76% lysis.
1 = 75% lysis.
2 = 50% lysis.
3 = 25% lysis.
4 = 0 lysis.

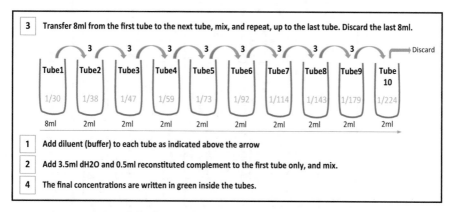

Fig. 10.2 Complement dilution for CFT

	1 (1/30)	2 (1/38)	3 (1/47)	4 (1/59)	5 (1/73)	6 (1/92)	7 (1/114)	8 (1/143)	9 (1/179)	10 (1/224)	11 control	12
A	1- 50ul buffer 2- 25ul from 1/30 diluted complement	1- 50ul buffer 2- 25ul from 1/38 diluted complement	1- 50ul buffer 2- 25ul from 1/38 diluted complement	1- 50ul buffer 2- 25ul from 1/59 diluted complement	1- 50ul buffer 2- 25ul from 1/73 diluted complement	1- 50ul buffer 2- 25ul from 1/92 diluted complement	1- 50ul buffer 2- 25ul from 1/114 diluted complement	1- 50ul buffer 2- 25ul from 1/143 diluted complement	1- 50ul buffer 2- 25ul from 1/179 diluted complement	1- 50ul buffer 2- 25ul from 1/224 diluted complement	1- 75ul buffer	
B	1- 50ul buffer 2- 25ul from 1/30 diluted complement	1- 50ul buffer 2- 25ul from 1/38 diluted complement	1- 50ul buffer 2- 25ul from 1/47 diluted complement	1- 50ul buffer 2- 25ul from 1/59 diluted complement	1- 50ul buffer 2- 25ul from 1/73 diluted complement	1- 50ul buffer 2- 25ul from 1/92 diluted complement	1- 50ul buffer 2- 25ul from 1/114 diluted complement	1- 50ul buffer 2- 25ul from 1/143 diluted complement	1- 50ul buffer 2- 25ul from 1/179 diluted complement	11- 50ul buffer 2- 25ul from 1/224 diluted complement	1- 75ul buffer	
C	1- 50ul buffer 2- 25ul from 1/30 diluted complement	1- 50ul buffer 2- 25ul from 1/38 diluted complement	1- 50ul buffer 2- 25ul from 1/47 diluted complement	1- 50ul buffer 2- 25ul from 1/59 diluted complement	1- 50ul buffer 2- 25ul from 1/73 diluted complement	1- 50ul buffer 2- 25ul from 1/92 diluted complement	1- 50ul buffer 2- 25ul from 1/114 diluted complement	1- 50ul buffer 2- 25ul from 1/143 diluted complement	1- 50ul buffer 2- 25ul from 1/179 diluted complement	1- 50ul buffer 2- 25ul from 1/224 diluted complement	1- 75ul buffer	
D	1- 50ul buffer 2- 25ul from 1/30 diluted complement	1- 50ul buffer 2- 25ul from 1/38 diluted complement	1- 50ul buffer 2- 25ul from 1/47 diluted complement	1- 50ul buffer 2- 25ul from 1/59 diluted complement	1- 50ul buffer 2- 25ul from 1/73 diluted complement	1- 50ul buffer 2- 25ul from 1/92 diluted complement	1- 50ul buffer 2- 25ul from 1/114 diluted complement	1- 50ul buffer 2- 25ul from 1/143 diluted complement	1- 50ul buffer 2- 25ul from 1/179 diluted complement	1- 50ul buffer 2- 25ul from 1/224 diluted complement	1- 75ul buffer	
E	1- 50ul buffer 2- 25ul from 1/30 diluted complement	1- 50ul buffer 2- 25ul from 1/38 diluted complement	1- 50ul buffer 2- 25ul from 1/47 diluted complement	1- 50ul buffer 2- 25ul from 1/59 diluted complement	1- 50ul buffer 2- 25ul from 1/73 diluted complement	1- 50ul buffer 2- 25ul from 1/92 diluted complement	1- 50ul buffer 2- 25ul from 1/114 diluted complement	1- 50ul buffer 2- 25ul from 1/143 diluted complement	1- 50ul buffer 2- 25ul from 1/179 diluted complement	1- 50ul buffer 2- 25ul from 1/224 diluted complement	1- 75ul buffer	
F	1- 50ul buffer 2- 25ul from 1/30 diluted complement	1- 50ul buffer 2- 25ul from 1/38 diluted complement	1- 50ul buffer 2- 25ul from 1/47 diluted complement	1- 50ul buffer 2- 25ul from 1/59 diluted complement	1- 50ul buffer 2- 25ul from 1/73 diluted complement	1- 50ul buffer 2- 25ul from 1/92 diluted complement	1- 50ul buffer 2- 25ul from 1/114 diluted complement	1- 50ul buffer 2- 25ul from 1/143 diluted complement	1- 50ul buffer 2- 25ul from 1/179 diluted complement	1- 50ul buffer 2- 25ul from 1/224 diluted complement	1- 75ul buffer	
G												

Fig. 10.3   Setting up complement titration

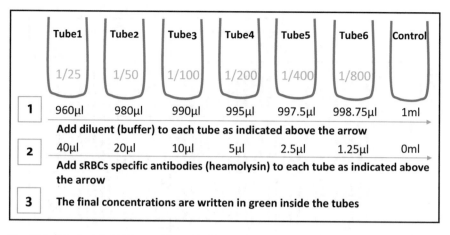

Fig. 10.4 Dilution of sRBCs-specific antibodies (hemolysin)

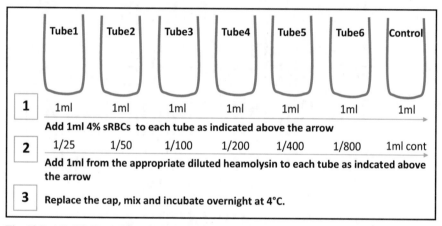

Fig. 10.5 4% sRBCs with hemolysin preparation

8. To determine the optimal sensitizing concentration (OSC) of the sensitized sRBCs, find the dilution that shows the most lysis with the highest dilution.
9. To determine a hemolytic dose giving 50% lysis (HDSO) of complement, find within the OSC of hemolysin the dilution that shows 50% lysis (score = 2).

Example
In the example in Fig. 10.7 the OSC is 1/100, and the HDSO is 1/114; however, the complement is used at 3HDSO, which in this example is equal to $1/114 \times 3 = 1/3$.

Standard Antigen Preparation [1]

Newly purchased standard antigens with new bath numbers must be titered. Therefore, six dilutions have to be selected to test the new antigen batch, as suggested on the antigen vial. For instance, if the optimal dilution suggested on the

	1/30	1/38	1/47	1/59	1/73	1/92	1/114	1/143	1/179	1/224	control	
	1	2	3	4	5	6	7	8	9	10	11	12
A	4- add 25ul from the sensitized SRBCs that were prepared from 1/25 diluted heamolysin	4- add 25ul from the sensitized SRBCs that were prepared from 1/25 diluted heamolysin	4- add 25ul from the sensitized SRBCs that were prepared from 1/25 diluted heamolysin	4- add 25ul from the sensitized SRBCs that were prepared from 1/25 diluted heamolysin	4- add 25ul from the sensitized SRBCs that were prepared from 1/25 diluted heamolysin	4- add 25ul from the sensitized SRBCs that were prepared from 1/25 diluted heamolysin	4- add 25ul from the sensitized SRBCs that were prepared from 1/25 diluted heamolysin	4- add 25ul from the sensitized SRBCs that were prepared from 1/25 diluted heamolysin	4- add 25ul from the sensitized SRBCs that were prepared from 1/25 diluted heamolysin	4- add 25ul from the sensitized SRBCs that were prepared from 1/25 diluted heamolysin	4- add 25ul from the sensitized SRBCs that were prepared from 1/25 diluted heamolysin	
B	4- add 25ul from the sensitized SRBCs that were prepared from 1/50 diluted heamolysin	4- add 25ul from the sensitized SRBCs that were prepared from 1/50 diluted heamolysin	4- add 25ul from the sensitized SRBCs that were prepared from 1/50 diluted heamolysin	4- add 25ul from the sensitized SRBCs that were prepared from 1/50 diluted heamolysin	4- add 25ul from the sensitized SRBCs that were prepared from 1/50 diluted heamolysin	4- add 25ul from the sensitized SRBCs that were prepared from 1/50 diluted heamolysin	4- add 25ul from the sensitized SRBCs that were prepared from 1/50 diluted heamolysin	4- add 25ul from the sensitized SRBCs that were prepared from 1/50 diluted heamolysin	4- add 25ul from the sensitized SRBCs that were prepared from 1/50 diluted heamolysin	4- add 25ul from the sensitized SRBCs that were prepared from 1/50 diluted heamolysin	4- add 25ul from the sensitized SRBCs that were prepared from 1/50 diluted heamolysin	
C	4- add 25ul from the sensitized SRBCs that were prepared from 1/100 diluted heamolysin	4- add 25ul from the sensitized SRBCs that were prepared from 1/100 diluted heamolysin	4- add 25ul from the sensitized SRBCs that were prepared from 1/100 diluted heamolysin	4- add 25ul from the sensitized SRBCs that were prepared from 1/100 diluted heamolysin	4- add 25ul from the sensitized SRBCs that were prepared from 1/100 diluted heamolysin	4- add 25ul from the sensitized SRBCs that were prepared from 1/100 diluted heamolysin	4- add 25ul from the sensitized SRBCs that were prepared from 1/100 diluted heamolysin	4- add 25ul from the sensitized SRBCs that were prepared from 1/100 diluted heamolysin	4- add 25ul from the sensitized SRBCs that were prepared from 1/100 diluted heamolysin	4- add 25ul from the sensitized SRBCs that were prepared from 1/100 diluted heamolysin	4- add 25ul from the sensitized SRBCs that were prepared from 1/100 diluted heamolysin	
D	4- add 25ul from the sensitized SRBCs that were prepared from 1/200 diluted heamolysin	4- add 25ul from the sensitized SRBCs that were prepared from 1/200 diluted heamolysin	4- add 25ul from the sensitized SRBCs that were prepared from 1/200 diluted heamolysin	4- add 25ul from the sensitized SRBCs that were prepared from 1/200 diluted heamolysin	4- add 25ul from the sensitized SRBCs that were prepared from 1/200 diluted heamolysin	4- add 25ul from the sensitized SRBCs that were prepared from 1/200 diluted heamolysin	4- add 25ul from the sensitized SRBCs that were prepared from 1/200 diluted heamolysin	4- add 25ul from the sensitized SRBCs that were prepared from 1/200 diluted heamolysin	4- add 25ul from the sensitized SRBCs that were prepared from 1/200 diluted heamolysin	4- add 25ul from the sensitized SRBCs that were prepared from 1/200 diluted heamolysin	4- add 25ul from the sensitized SRBCs that were prepared from 1/200 diluted heamolysin	
E	4- add 25ul from the sensitized SRBCs that were prepared from 1/400 diluted heamolysin	4- add 25ul from the sensitized SRBCs that were prepared from 1/400 diluted heamolysin	4- add 25ul from the sensitized SRBCs that were prepared from 1/400 diluted heamolysin	4- add 25ul from the sensitized SRBCs that were prepared from 1/400 diluted heamolysin	4- add 25ul from the sensitized SRBCs that were prepared from 1/400 diluted heamolysin	4- add 25ul from the sensitized SRBCs that were prepared from 1/400 diluted heamolysin	4- add 25ul from the sensitized SRBCs that were prepared from 1/400 diluted heamolysin	4- add 25ul from the sensitized SRBCs that were prepared from 1/400 diluted heamolysin	4- add 25ul from the sensitized SRBCs that were prepared from 1/400 diluted heamolysin	4- add 25ul from the sensitized SRBCs that were prepared from 1/400 diluted heamolysin	4- add 25ul from the sensitized SRBCs that were prepared from 1/400 diluted heamolysin	
F	4- add 25ul from the sensitized SRBCs that were prepared from 1/800 diluted heamolysin	4- add 25ul from the sensitized SRBCs that were prepared from 1/800 diluted heamolysin	4- add 25ul from the sensitized SRBCs that were prepared from 1/800 diluted heamolysin	4- add 25ul from the sensitized SRBCs that were prepared from 1/800 diluted heamolysin	4- add 25ul from the sensitized SRBCs that were prepared from 1/800 diluted heamolysin	4- add 25ul from the sensitized SRBCs that were prepared from 1/800 diluted heamolysin	4- add 25ul from the sensitized SRBCs that were prepared from 1/800 diluted heamolysin	4- add 25ul from the sensitized SRBCs that were prepared from 1/800 diluted heamolysin	4- add 25ul from the sensitized SRBCs that were prepared from 1/800 diluted heamolysin	4- add 25ul from the sensitized SRBCs that were prepared from 1/800 diluted heamolysin	4- add 25ul from the sensitized SRBCs that were prepared from 1/800 diluted heamolysin	
G	4- add 25ul from the sensitized SRBCs control	4- add 25ul from the sensitized SRBCs control	4- add 25ul from the sensitized SRBCs control	4- add 25ul from the sensitized SRBCs control	4- add 25ul from the sensitized SRBCs control	4- add 25ul from the sensitized SRBCs control	4- add 25ul from the sensitized SRBCs control	4- add 25ul from the sensitized SRBCs control	4- add 25ul from the sensitized SRBCs control	4- add 25ul from the sensitized SRBCs control	4- add 25ul from the sensitized SRBCs control	

Fig. 10.6 Addition of sensitized sRBCs to the microtiter plate

| Heamolysin | Complement |||||||||||
	1/30	1/38	1/47	1/59	1/73	1/92	1/114	1/143	1/179	1/224	Control
1/25	0	0	Tr	1	2	3	4	4	4	4	4
1/50	0	0	0	Tr	1	2	3	4	4	4	4
1/100	0	0	0	0	Tr	1	2	4	4	4	4
1/200	0	0	0	Tr	1	2	4	4	4	4	4
1/400	0	0	0	Tr	1	2	4	4	4	4	4
1/800	0	Tr	1	2	4	4	4	4	4	4	4
control	4	4	4	4	4	4	4	4	4	4	4

Fig. 10.7 Scoring example of complement and sensitized sRBC preparation

antigen vial is 1:40, then select 1:10, 1:20, 1:30, 1:40, 1:50, and 1:60 with a total volume of at least 600 µl to determine the optimal dilution of the standard A, two microtiter plates are needed.

First plate,

1. This plate is used as positive and negative antisera controls and C back titration. The antiserum is diluted 1/16 and incubated at 56 °C for 30 min as an inactivation step.
2. Add 25 µl of buffer into columns 2–5, rows A–F, and 50 µl of buffer into wells on column 6, rows A–F.
3. Add 25 µl from the appropriate antiserum into columns 1, 2, and 6, and double dilute from columns 2 to 5.
4. Add 25 µl of appropriate antigen dilution into wells on columns 1–5, rows A–F.
5. Add 25 µl of 3HDSO complement to columns 1–6, rows A–F.
6. Mix by tapping the plate and incubate overnight at 4 °C.

For the complement C' back titration.

1. Add 25 µl buffer and 25 µl from the appropriate antigen dilution into the following wells, columns 10–12, rows A–F.
2. Mix by tapping the plate.
3. Add 25 µl 3HDSO complement into columns 10, rows A–F, 25 µl 1HDSO into column 11, rows A–F, and 25 µl of 1/2HDSO complement into column 12, rows A–F.

Second plate,

1. This plate is done on the positive and negative samples of a patient's specimen. The serum is diluted 1/16 and incubated at 56 °C for 30 min as an inactivation step.
2. The same procedure done with the positive antiserum control (first plate) is done for both specimens. However, 25 µl of 3HDSO complements is added to all wells (columns 1–12, rows A–H).
3. Mix by tapping the plate and incubate overnight at 4 °C.

The following steps are common between the first and the second microtiter plates:

1. After the overnight incubation, incubate the plates for 30 min at 37 °C, and incubate 4% sensitized sRBCs at 37 °C for 30 min as well.
2. Add 25 µl of sensitized sRBCs, and incubate for 30 min at 37 °C, mixing the plates by tapping at 10, 20, and at the end of the incubation time 30 min.
3. Centrifuge to settle the cells.
4. Read the plates.

   Note: The dilution where positive antiserum control provides the highest titer and the predetermined titer for a positive sample is the optimal dilution of antigen. Moreover, the test must show a regular complement back titration pattern and the negative samples should show negative results.

Positive Control and Antisera Preparation [1]

Titration must be done on all new antisera batches, and as instructed by the manufacturers. For instance, if the manufacturers suggest 1:40 to be the optimal dilution of antisera, then perform a series of dilution that includes 1:20, 1:30, 1:35, 1:40, 1:45, 1:50, 1:55, and 1:60 diluted in buffer in a total volume of at least 600 µl.
   Follow the steps listed below and illustrated in Fig. 10.8

1. From the appropriate antisera dilution, add 50 µl into column 1, and 25 µl buffer into wells on columns 2–6, rows A–H.
2. Make twofold dilution from the antisera, as shown in Fig. 10.8.
3. Add 25 µl of antigens at its working dilution.
4. Add 25 µl of the appropriate HD50 complement as Fig. 10.8 shows.
5. Mix by tapping the plate and incubate at 4 °C overnight.

   Note: Wells 7–9 represent the antigens back-titration, whereas wells 10–12 represent the complement back titration.

6. After incubation, incubate the plate at 37 °C for 30 min. Meanwhile, prepare the sufficient amount of sensitized sRBCs by incubating it at 37 °C for 30 min.
7. Add 25 µl of sensitized sRBCs, and incubate at 37 °C for 30 min with mixing every 10 min.
8. Centrifuge to settle the cells and read the results.

   Dilution that shows complete fixation at the highest antisera dilution is the optimal dilution to be used with antisera. At this step, all the reagents required for CFT are prepared.

	1	2	3	4	5	6	7	8	9	10	11	12
A	1- add 50ul of 1/20 diluted antisera 2- Transfer 25ul to well 2A	1- add 25ul buffer 2- Transfer 25ul to well 3A.	1- add 25ul buffer 2- Transfer 25ul to well 4A.	1- add 25ul buffer 2- Transfer 25ul to well 5A.	1- add 25ul buffer 2- Discard 25ul from this well	1- add 25ul buffer 2- add 25ul of appropriate serum control.	1- add 25ul buffer 4- add 25ul 3HD50 complement	1- add 25ul buffer 1HD50 complement	1- add 25ul buffer 4- add 25ul 1/5HD50 complement	1- add 50ul buffer 4- add 25ul 3HD50 complement	1- add 50ul buffer 4- add 25ul 1HD50 complement	1- add 50ul buffer 4- add 25ul 1/5HD50 complement
B	1- add 50ul of 1/30 diluted antisera 2- Transfer 25ul to well 2B.	1- add 25ul buffer 2- Transfer 25ul to well 3B.	1- add 25ul buffer 2- Transfer 25ul to well 4B.	1- add 25ul buffer 2- Transfer 25ul to well 5B.	1- add 25ul buffer 2- Discard 25ul from this well	1- add 25ul buffer 2- add 25ul of appropriate serum control.						
C	1- add 50ul of 1/35 diluted antisera 2- Transfer 25ul to well 2C	1- add 25ul buffer 2- Transfer 25ul to well 3C.	1- add 25ul buffer 2- Transfer 25ul to well 4C.	1- add 25ul buffer 2- Transfer 25ul to well 5C.	1- add 25ul buffer 2- Discard 25ul from this well	1- add 25ul buffer 2- add 25ul of appropriate serum control.						
D	1- add 50ul of 1/40 diluted antisera 2- Transfer 25ul to well 2D.	1- add 25ul buffer 2- Transfer 25ul to well 3D.	1- add 25ul buffer 2- Transfer 25ul to well 4D.	1- add 25ul buffer 2- Transfer 25ul to well 5D.	1- add 25ul buffer 2- Discard 25ul from this well	1- add 25ul buffer 2- add 25ul of appropriate serum control.						
E	1- add 50ul of 1/45 diluted antisera 2- Transfer 25ul to well 2E.	1- add 25ul buffer 2- Transfer 25ul to well 3E.	1- add 25ul buffer 2- Transfer 25ul to well 4E.	1- add 25ul buffer 2- Transfer 25ul to well 5E	1- add 25ul buffer 2- Discard 25ul from this well	1- add 25ul buffer 2- add 25ul of appropriate serum control.						
F	1- add 50ul of 1/50 diluted antisera 2- Transfer 25ul to well 2F.	1- add 25ul buffer 2- Transfer 25ul to well 3F.	1- add 25ul buffer 2- Transfer 25ul to well 4F.	1- add 25ul buffer 2- Transfer 25ul to well 5F.	1- add 25ul buffer 2- Discard 25ul from this well	1- add 25ul buffer 2- add 25ul of appropriate serum control.						
G	1- add 50ul of 1/55 diluted antisera 2- Transfer 25ul to well 2G.	1- add 25ul buffer 2- Transfer 25ul to well 3G.	1- add 25ul buffer 2- Transfer 25ul to well 4G.	1- add 25ul buffer 2- Transfer 25ul to well 5G.	1- add 25ul buffer 2- Discard 25ul from this well	1- add 25ul buffer 2- add 25ul of appropriate serum control.						
H	1- add 50ul of 1/60 diluted antisera 2- Transfer 25ul to well 2H.	1- add 25ul buffer 2- Transfer 25ul to well 3H.	1- add 25ul buffer 2- Transfer 25ul to well 4H	1- add 25ul buffer 2- Transfer 25ul to well 5H.	1- add 25ul buffer 2- Discard 25ul from this well	1- add 25ul buffer 2- add 25ul of appropriate serum control.						

Fig. 10.8 Preparation of positive control and antisera

CFT Steps [1]

1. Pre-heat the 1/16 diluted patient serum at 56 °C for 30 min.

   Note: For 1/16 dilution add 50 µl of serum into 750 µl of buffer.

2. For steps 2–6 see Fig. 10.9.
3. Mix the reagent by tapping the plate, and then incubate at 4 °C overnight.

Controls must run together with the test such as antiserum control, antigen control, and complement control. The antisera control is done as shown in Fig. 10.9. As for antigen and complement controls, see the steps listed below:

1. For antigen control add 25 µl of buffer to row B, and 25 µl from the antigen and mix by tapping the plate. Subsequently, add 25 µl 3HD50 complement, and mix by tapping the plate.
2. For the complement control, add 25 µl of 3HD50 complement to well 10A, 25 µl of 1HD50 complement to well 11A, and 25 µl of 1/2HD50 complement to well 12A, and then add 50 µl of buffer to all three wells.
3. Incubate overnight at 4 °C.

Note: For any component omitted, add 25 µl of buffer to have a final volume of 4×25 µl.

4. Incubate the plate with sensitized sRBCs for 30 min at 37 °C.
5. Add 25 µl of sensitized sRBCs to all wells and mix.
6. Incubate the plate at 37 °C for 30 min, and mix by tapping the plate every 10 min.
7. Incubate the plate at 4 °C for 2 h and read the results after a 10-min incubation period on the bench.

Results Interpretation [1]

Figure 10.10 is an example explaining the process of reading CFT results for viral infection.

Some of the problems that might be associated with CFT results include:

1. Lack of lysis in serum control wells where only serum, complement, and sensitized sRBCs are present indicates that the patient serum possesses anti-complementary activating antibodies; therefore, guinea pig serum should be used to treat the issue.
2. The presence of anti-hemagglutination activating antibodies in patient sera requires the use of sRBCs to treat the sera.
3. Complete lysis, 50% lysis, and no lysis should be seen with 3HD50 complement, 1HD50 complement, and 1/2HD50 complement respectively, with both antigen and complement back titration wells.

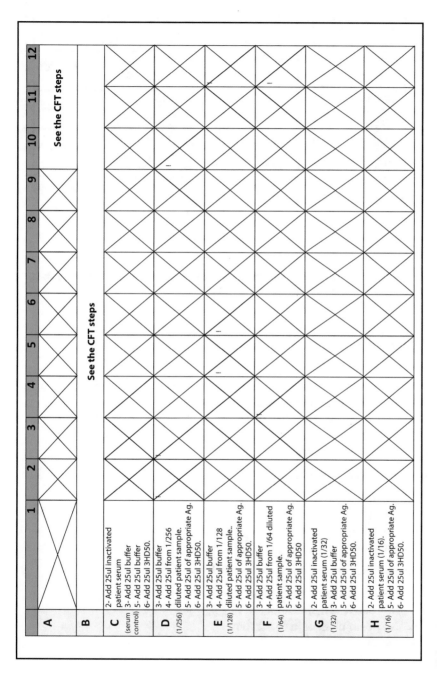

Fig. 10.9 CFT steps

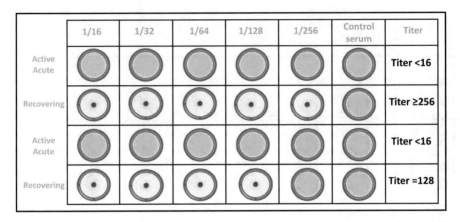

Fig. 10.10 An example of CFT results

Reference

1. Coleman PN. Standardization of the Wassermann test using preserved complement titrated to 50 per cent haemolysis. Br J Vener Dis. 1952;28(3):129–37.

Study Questions

1. **CFT is used to:**

   (a) **Measure specific antibodies in patient serum**.
   (b) Measure hormone levels in patient's serum.
   (c) Detect pregnancy.
   (d) Detect genetic diseases.

2. **A patient's serum contains:**

   (a) Antibodies.
   (b) Antigens.
   (c) Complements.
   (d) **All the above**.

3. **Patient serum must be heated before CFT to:**

   (a) Destroy antibodies in the serum.
   (b) Destroy antigens in the serum.
   (c) **Destroy complement in the serum**.
   (d) All the above.

4. **Patient serum, in CFT, containing specific antibodies of interest binds to_____and fix_____ on the surface of antibodies:**

    (a) Antibodies and complement.
    (b) Antigens and antibodies.
    (c) **Antigens and complement**.
    (d) Complement and complement.

5. **In CFT, in positive patient serum with specific antibodies of interest the:**

    (a) sRBCs sensitized with specific antigens are completely lysed.
    (b) sRBCs sensitized with specific antigens are 50% lysed.
    (c) sRBCs sensitized with specific antigens are 70% lysed.
    (d) **sRBCs sensitized with specific antigens are not lysed.**

6. **In CFT, in negative patient serum the:**

    (a) **sRBCs sensitized with specific antigens are lysed.**
    (b) sRBCs sensitized with specific antigens are not lysed.
    (c) sRBCs sensitized with specific antigens are 50% lysed.
    (d) None of the above.

7. **CFT requires:**

    (a) **Sensitized sRBCs**.
    (b) Slide test.
    (c) Gel.
    (d) None of the above.

8. **The titer of the below CFT is:**

    (a) <16.
    (b) >256.
    (c) **1/128**.
    (d) 1/32.

| 1/16 | 1/32 | 1/64 | 1/128 | 1/256 | control |

Chapter 11
Radioimmunoassay (RIA)

Learning Objectives
By the end of this chapter the reader should be able to:

1. Describe the principle of RIA.
2. List the reagents required for the RIA test.
3. List the general steps performed during the RIA test.
4. Understand the steps and calculation required to interpret RIA test results.

Yalow and Berson first introduced **Radioimmunoassay (RIA)** in 1959 [1]. RIA users are recommended to determine if the samples they are utilizing need to be cleaned by **ion exchange chromatography** and **freeze drying/lyophilization** [2]. The cleaning process serves to concentrate the analyte, especially when the assay sensitivity and the amount of the analyte to be measured are low [2]. RIA is a technique that quantifies the amount of specific antigen in a patient sample [2, 3]. The technique requires the use of radioisotopes such as ^{125}I, which has safety concerns and a short shelf life; therefore, the radioisotope used in RIA was modified and replaced by enzyme-generating enzyme immunoassay (ELA) and enzyme-linked immunosorbent assay (ELISA) [2, 3].

Radioimmunoassay (RIA)

Principle

Radioimmunoassay is a quantitative test for detecting specific antigens in patient serum. In this assay, the sample antigen is incubated with its complementary antibodies allowing them to bind [2–4]. Subsequently, the added radioactive labeled antigen competes with sample antigens [2–4]. A secondary antibody specific to the complementary antibodies is added to bind with the complementary antibodies and form complexes that participate at the bottom of the well, separating the

© Springer International Publishing AG, part of Springer Nature 2018
R. Y. Alhabbab, *Basic Serological Testing*, Techniques in Life Science and
Biomedicine for the Non-Expert, https://doi.org/10.1007/978-3-319-77694-1_11

complementary antibodies from the solution [2–4]. Subsequently, centrifugation forms a pellet containing sample antigens, radioactive antigens, complementary antibodies, and secondary antibodies [2–4]. The concentration of the sample anti-gens can then be determined by measuring the radioactivity of the pallet; therefore, the more sample antigen present in the sample, the less radiation is obtained (Fig. 11.1) [2–4].

Note: Some kits provide tubes coated with secondary antibodies.

RIA Reagents

1. Buffer.
2. Standard: antigens similar to the target antigen in patient samples usually comes in several vials with known concentrations [4, 5].
3. Rabbit antibodies specific for the tested antigens (complementary antibodies).
4. Radioactively labeled antigens (antigens similar to test antigen in patient serum) called **tracer** [4].
5. Secondary antibodies specific to the complementary antibodies (goat anti-rabbit IgG). Some kits provide tubes coated with the secondary antibodies [4].
6. Controls (positive and negative).

RIA Steps [4, 5]

All amounts, incubation times and centrifugation speed must be in accordance with the manufacturer's instruction.

1. Add the complementary antibodies to labeled tubes (in duplicate) that contain the standards, controls, and samples.
2. After incubation, add the tracer to the reaction and incubate.
3. Add secondary antibodies and incubate (except for total count (TC) tubes).
4. Add the recommended amount of buffer (except for TC tubes) and centrifuge.
5. Aspirate the supernatant (except for TC tubes).
6. Count using gamma counter and calculate the results.

Preparation of non-specific binding (NSB), total binding (TB), and total count (TC) tubes.

These three tubes must be associated with every test.

NSB

1. Add buffer to the NSB tube.
2. Add tracer to the NSB tube.
3. Incubate at 4 °C.
4. Add secondary antibodies to the NSB tube and incubate at room temperature.

Fig. 11.1 The principle of radioimmunoassay

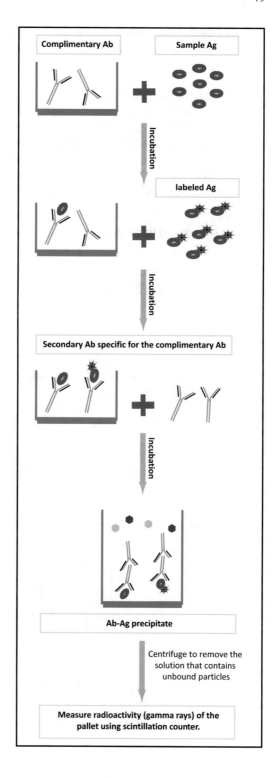

5. Add buffer to the NSB tube, centrifuge, and aspirate the supernatant.
6. Count and calculate the results.

TB

1. Add buffer to the TB tube.
2. Add complementary antibodies to the TB tube.
3. Incubate at 4 °C as instructed.
4. Add tracer to the TB tube and incubate at 4 °C.
5. Add secondary antibodies to the TB tube, incubate at room temperature, and centrifuge.
6. Aspirate the supernatant, count, and calculate the results.

TC tubes
    TC tubes contain tracer only.

RIA Results Interpretation

1. Using counts per minute (CPM), calculate the NSB and TB.
2. Calculate B_O from the following equation: $B_O = TB - NSB$ [4].
3. Calculate $B/B_O\%$ for standards and samples by using the following equation: $B/B_O\%$ = (average standard, unknown sample or control CPM – NSB)/$B_O \times 100$ [4].
4. Plot B/B_O % for standards versus the concentration of standard antigens (given by the manufacturer) using semi-logarithmic graph paper, as shown in Fig. 11.2 [4].
5. The unknown concentrations of samples and controls are determined by interpolation of their calculated B/B_O % from the standard concentration.

Fig. 11.2 Standard curve plot

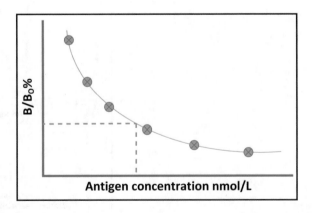

References

1. Annesley TM. It's about the journey, not the destination: the birth of radioimmunoassay. 1960. Clin Chem. 2010;56(4):671–2.
2. Grange RD, Thompson JP, Lambert DG. Radioimmunoassay, enzyme and non-enzyme-based immunoassays. Br J Anaesth. 2014;112(2):213–6.
3. Gan SD, Patel KR. Enzyme immunoassay and enzyme-linked immunosorbent assay. J Invest Dermatol. 2013;133(9):e12.
4. Institute of Isotopes Ltd. T4 [^{125}I] RIA KIT. Izotop. Available from: http://www.izotop.hu/pdf/immuno/rk11CT1_a.pdf. Accessed 7 September 2017.
5. Phoenix Pharmaceuticals, Inc. General protocol for radio immunoassay kit. Phoenix. Available from: http://www.phoenixbiotech.net/catalog/repository/QCdata_RIK/10-1280-color-RIA.pdf. Accessed 10 September 2017.

Study Questions

1. **Samples used for RIA are cleaned:**

   (a) Using chromatography.
   (b) To concentrate the analyte.
   (c) When the amount of the analyte is low.
   (d) **All the above**.

2. **The RIA test requires:**

   (a) **Radioisotopes**.
   (b) Enzyme.
   (c) Immunofluorescent materials.
   (d) Gold particles.

3. **RIA is replaced by:**

   (a) PCR.
   (b) **ELISA**.
   (c) Radial immunodiffusion.
   (d) Latex agglutination.

4. **RIA requires:**

   (a) **Radioisotope labeled antigens**.
   (b) Complementary antibodies (cAb) to antigens in patient serum.
   (c) Antibodies specific to cAb.
   (d) All the above.

5. **Each RIA test needs.**

   (a) NSB tubes.
   (b) TC tubes.
   (c) TB tubes.
   (d) **All the above**.

Chapter 12
Enzyme Immunoassay (EIAs) and Enzyme-Linked Immunosorbent Assay (ELISA)

Learning Objectives
By the end of this chapter the reader should be able to:

1. Describe the four ELISA principles.
2. List the reagents required for each ELISA test.
3. List the general steps performed for the different types of ELISA test.
4. Understand the steps and calculations required to interpret ELISA test results.

In 1971, the enzyme-linked immunosorbent assay (ELISA) was introduced by Engrail and Perlman, where they determined the concentrations of unknown specific antibodies by immobilizing antigens into a microplate well, and incubating antisera of the sample and antibodies conjugated to an enzyme with the antigens that are coating the microplate well [1, 2]. On the other hand, the enzyme immunoassay (EIA) was introduced independently by Van Weemen and Schuurs to measure antigen concentrations rather than antibodies [3]. However, the two terms (EIA and ELISA) are used interchangeably. There are four major principles for ELISA methods: **direct ELISA**, **indirect ELISA**, **sandwich ELISA** and **competitive ELISA**.

Enzyme-Linked Immunosorbent Assay (ELISA)

Principle

Direct ELISA

In general, all ELISAs are quantitative tests to determine the concentration of unknown specific antibodies or antigens. Direct ELISA requires the immobilization of patient antigens on a microplate well, and complementary antibodies to the

© Springer International Publishing AG, part of Springer Nature 2018
R. Y. Alhabbab, *Basic Serological Testing*, Techniques in Life Science and
Biomedicine for the Non-Expert, https://doi.org/10.1007/978-3-319-77694-1_12

patient antigens [2]. Complementary antibodies are conjugated to an enzyme that reacts with a substrate. The substrate is converted into detectable product after interacting with the enzyme [2] (Fig. 12.1).

Several advantages are associated with this method, such as simplicity and the requirement for less time than the other ELISA methods. However, the sensitivity of this method is low for two reasons. First, samples containing a large number of antigens other than the target one can be a problem, especially when the target antigen is present in a low concentration [2]. Moreover, complementary antibodies are attached to an enzyme that can influence their affinity, therefore reducing the sensitivity of the test [2].

Indirect ELISA

Like direct ELISAs, indirect ELISAs require the immobilization of patient antigens on the surface of microplate well [2]. However, an indirect ELISA uses two types of antibodies instead of one. The first is primary antibodies, which are complementary and specific to the patient antigen, and form complexes with the patient antigen on the surface of the microplate well [2]. The second antibodies are specific to the Fc region of the primary antibodies, and conjugated to an enzyme that reacts with a substrate to produce detectable products (Fig. 12.2) [2].

This method is more sensitive than direct ELISA because it uses secondary antibodies. However, the method has the same issue of having complex and a large number of antigens other than the target antigen in patient serum [2].

Sandwich ELISA

With this method, unlike direct and indirect ELISAs, specific antibodies (called capture antibodies or complementary antibodies) to the antigen of interest are adsorbed to the microplate well. Therefore, the sandwich ELISA overcomes the issue of reduced sensitivity that is associated with both direct and indirect ELISA owing to various proteins that could be adsorbed onto the microplate well. Patient antigens bind to capture antibodies, and secondary antibodies, conjugate to an enzyme (called conjugate) and specific to the patient antigen, binds to the patient antigens that are on the capture antibodies. Finally, the enzyme conjugated to secondary antibodies reacts with the added substrate to produce detectable products (Fig. 12.3).

This method uses two specific antibodies, which increase its sensitivity and cost compared to direct and indirect ELISA.

Fig. 12.1 Direct
enzyme-linked
immunosorbent assay
(ELISA) principle

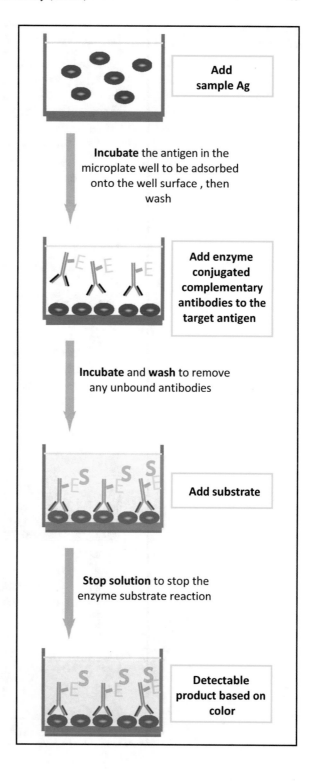

Fig. 12.2 Indirect ELISA principle

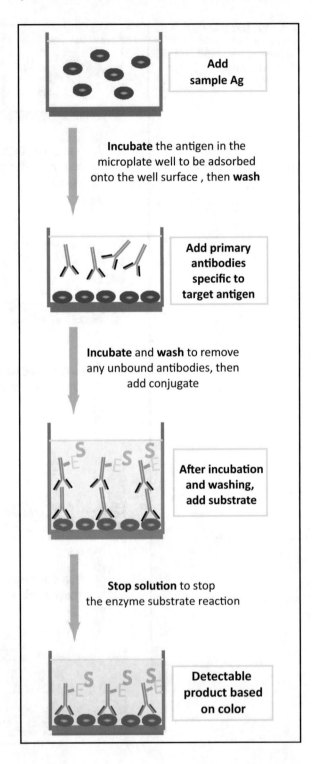

Fig. 12.3 Sandwich
ELISA principle

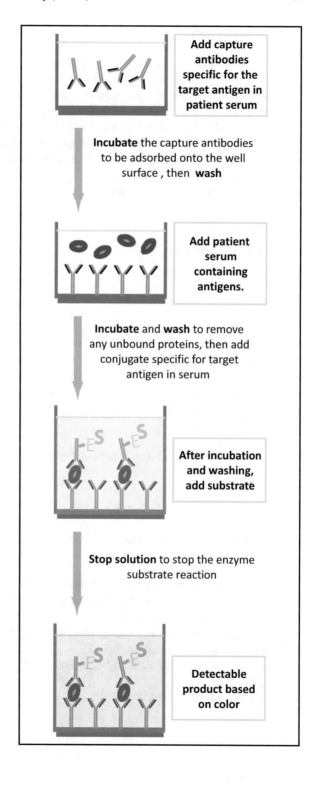

Competitive ELISA

This method depends on the competition between two antigens for binding on limited available antibodies site. The first antigen is the patient antigen, while the second one is usually similar to that antigen in patient serum but labeled with biotin or directly labeled with an enzyme. Here, the antigens compete for the same binding sites on the antibodies, and the number of antigens in the sample is inversely proportional to the level of signals generated. Biotinylated antigen binds to streptavidin, which can be labeled using several methods [2, 4]. The latter methods can generate different detectable products such as a change in color, induction of fluorescence, or chemiluminescence (Fig. 12.4).

ELISA Reagents and Steps

Direct ELISA

Reagents

1. Microtiter plate.
2. Patient serum that may contain the target antigens.
3. Controls.
4. Standards containing the target antigens with known concentrations.
5. Antibodies conjugated to an enzyme and specific to the patient antigens.
6. Substrate solution.
7. Stop solution.
8. Plate reader (read absorbance = optical density).

Steps

1. Coat the plate well with antigens of interest using the patient sample and standard antigens [5].
2. Incubate overnight at 4 °C.
3. Wash the plate three times with appropriate buffer and block the remaining protein binding site in the well by using blocking buffer and incubate, then wash again three times with buffer [5].
4. Add conjugate antibodies according to the manufacturer's instructions and incubate for 1–2 h at room temperature [5].
5. Wash the plate three times with buffer and add the substrate, as suggested by manufacturer.
6. Add stop solution and read the results.

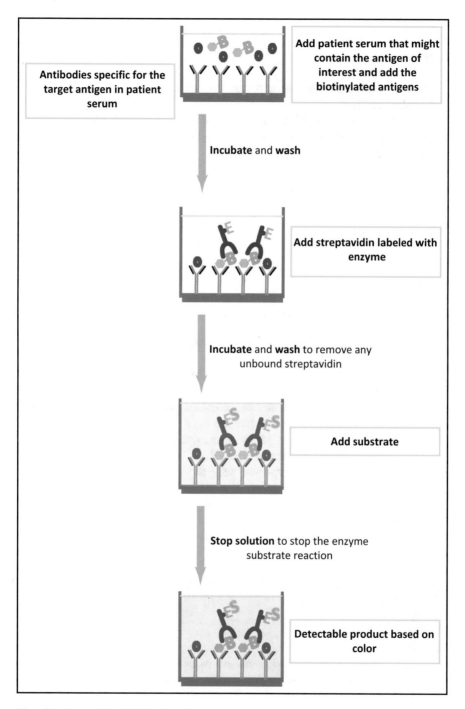

Fig. 12.4 Competitive ELISA principle

Indirect ELISA

Reagents

1. Patient sample that may contain the antigens of interest.
2. Standard antigens.
3. Primary antibodies specific to the antigen of interest in patient serum.
4. Secondary antibodies conjugated to an enzyme and specific to the Fc region of the primary antibodies.
5. Controls.
6. Substrate solution.
7. Stop solution.
8. Plate reader.
9. Microtiter plate.

Steps

1. Coat the microtiter plate well with antigens found in patient serum and standard antigens [6].
2. Incubate and wash three times with appropriate buffer as suggested by the manufacturer.
3. Block the remaining protein-binding site in the well using blocking buffer and wash three times with buffer [6].
4. Add primary antibodies, incubate, and wash as suggested by the manufacturer [6].
5. Add secondary antibodies (some kits use only secondary antibodies conjugate specific for the target antigens without using detection antibodies), incubate, and wash as suggested by the manufacturer [6].
6. Add substrate, incubate, and add stop solution as instructed by the manufacturer.

Sandwich ELISA

Reagents

1. Capture antibodies specific to the antigen of interest in patient serum.
2. Blocking solution.
3. Patient serum.
4. Standard antigens.
5. Microtiter plate.
6. Detection antibodies specific to antigens of interest in patient serum.
7. Secondary antibodies conjugated to an enzyme and specific to detection antibodies.
8. Substrate solution.
9. Stop solution.
10. Plate reader.

Steps

1. Coat the microtiter plate well with primary antibodies specific to patient antigens, incubate, and wash three times with appropriate buffer as suggested by the manufacturer [7].
2. Block the remaining protein-binding site in the well using blocking buffer and wash three times with buffer [7].
3. Add sample and standard antigens to the appropriate wells, incubate, and wash, as indicated by the manufacturer.
4. Add detection antibodies, incubate, and wash, as suggested by the manufacturer [7].
5. Add secondary antibodies, incubate, and wash, as indicated by the manufacturer [7].
6. Add substrate, incubate, and then add the stop solution, without washing.
7. Read the results.

Competitive ELISA

Reagents

1. Microtiter plate.
2. Antibodies specific to the antigen of interest in patient serum.
3. An antigen similar to the antigens of interest in the patient sample, but conjugated to an enzyme.
4. Standard antigens.
5. Blocking solution.
6. Substrate.
7. Stop solution.
8. Plate reader.

Steps

1. Coat the microtiter plate well with antibodies specific to the antigens of interest in patient serum, incubate, and wash three times with an appropriate buffer, as suggested by the manufacturer.
2. Block the remaining protein-binding sites in wells using blocking buffer and wash three times with buffer.
3. Add patient serum and standard antigens and conjugate to appropriate wells, incubate, and wash, as indicated by the manufacturer [2, 4].
4. Add substrate, incubate, and add stop solution, without washing.
5. Read the results.

In general, the most commonly used detection enzyme system in ELISAs is enzyme horseradish peroxidase (HRP) and its substrate alkaline phosphatase (ALP).

ELISA Results Interpretation

1. ELISA samples and standards must always be run in duplicate or triplicate, and the average absorbance must be calculated from the duplicate or triplicate and should be within 20% of the mean.
2. Including a standard curve is recommended for each ELISA plate by plotting the mean absorbance on the *x*-axis for every standard concentration versus the protein concentrations (provided by the manufacturer) on the *y*-axis. Subsequently, join the points in the graph to obtain the best-fit curve (Fig. 12.5a) [8].

Fig. 12.5 Standard curve graph of an ELISA

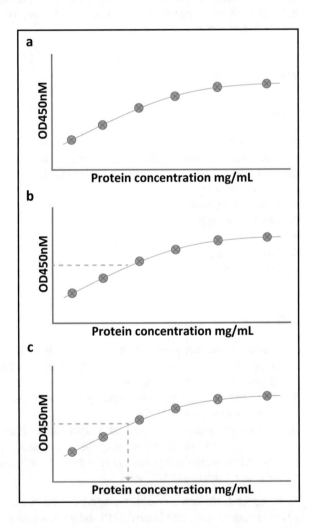

3. To determine the sample protein concentration, using the standard curve draw a horizontal line out of the y-axis from the mean absorbance value of the sample to reach the standard curve, as shown in Fig. 12.5b [8].
4. From the point of intersection, drop a second vertical line to the x-axis, as illustrated in Fig. 12.5c [8].
5. Record the protein concentration results.

Note: The value of the sample with very high protien concentration that is out of the detectable range must be diluted and after obtaining the reading, results must be multiplied by the dilution factor. Moreover, the coefficient of variation (CV) of the results must be no more than 2%.

References

1. Engvall E, Perlmann P. Enzyme-linked immunosorbent assay (ELISA). Quantitative assay of immunoglobulin G. Immunochemistry. 1971;8(9):871–4.
2. Grange RD, Thompson JP, Lambert DG. Radioimmunoassay, enzyme and non-enzyme-based immunoassays. Br J Anaesth. 2014;112(2):213–6.
3. Van Weemen BK, Schuurs AH. Immunoassay using antibody—enzyme conjugates. FEBS Lett. 1974;43(2):215–8.
4. Bhandari SS, Davies JE, Struck J, Ng LL. Influence of confounding factors on plasma mid-regional pro-adrenomedullin and mid-regional pro-A-type natriuretic peptide concentrations in healthy individuals. Biomarkers. 2011;16(3):281–7.
5. Bioss Antibodies. Direct ELISA protocol. Shopify. Available from: https://cdn.shopify.com/s/files/1/1223/3460/files/bioss_direct_elisa_protocol.pdf?11888709488737540494.   Accessed 16 September 2017.
6. Abcam discover more. Indirect ELISA Protocol. Abcam. 2016. Available from: http://www.abcam.com/ps/pdf/protocols/indirect%20elisa%20protocol.pdf. Accessed 16 September 2017.
7. Abcam discover more. Sandwich ELISA Protocol. Abcam. 2016. Available from: http://www.abcam.com/ps/pdf/protocols/sandwich_elisa.pdf. Accessed 16 September 2017.
8. Abcam. Calculating and Evaluating ELISA Data. Abcam. 2016. Available from: http://docs.abcam.com/pdf/protocols/calculating-and-evaluating-elisa-data.pdf. Accessed 17 September 2017

Study Questions

1. **ELISA is used to determine the concentrations of:**

   (a) **Specific antibodies or antigens.**
   (b) Specific antibodies only.
   (c) Specific antigens only.
   (d) None of the above.

2. **The principle of an ELISA can be:**

   (a) Direct.
   (b) Indirect.

(c) Sandwich.

(d) **All the above**.

3. **Direct ELISA requires:**

   (a) Immobilization of commercially provided antibodies specific to the target antigens in patient serum.

   (b) **One antibody specific to the target antigen and labeled with an enzyme**.

   (c) Primary antibodies specific to the target antigen and secondary antibodies specific to Fc region of primary antibodies and labeled with enzyme.

   (d) Detection antibodies specific to the target antigen and capture antibodies.

4. **Indirect ELISA requires:**

   (a) Immobilization of commercially provided antibodies specific to the target antigens in patient serum.

   (b) One antibody specific to the target antigen and labeled with an enzyme.

   (c) **Primary antibodies specific to the target antigen and secondary antibodies specific to the Fc region of primary antibodies and labeled with an enzyme**.

   (d) Detection antibodies specific to target antigen and capture antibodies.

5. **Direct ELISA is less sensitive than indirect ELISA because:**

   (a) Direct ELISA contains a large number of antigens other than the target one, whereas an indirect ELISA contains the target antigen only.

   (b) **Direct ELISA uses one primary antibody, whereas an indirect ELISA uses two antibodies**.

   (c) Direct ELISA uses detection and capture antibodies.

   (d) None of the above.

6. **Direct and indirect ELISAs are less sensitive than sandwich ELISAs because:**

   (a) **Large numbers of antigens other than the target one are immobilized to the reaction well**.

   (b) Only the target antigen is immobilized to the reaction well.

   (c) Specific antibodies are immobilized into the reaction well.

   (d) None of the above.

7. **Sandwich ELISA uses:**

   (a) Capture antibodies specific to the target antigen.

   (b) Detection antibodies specific to the target antigen.

   (c) Secondary antibodies specific to detection antibodies.

   (d) **All the above**.

8. **Competitive ELISAs depend on:**

   (a) **Competition between two antigens**.

   (b) Competition between two complements.

(c) Competition between enzymes.

(d) None of the above.

9. **ELISA results require:**

(a) **A standard curve**.

(b) An electromagnetic field.

(c) A microscope.

(d) All the above.

Chapter 13
Pregnancy Test

Learning Objectives
By the end of this chapter the reader should be able to:

1. Discuss the process of human chronic gonadotropin (hCG) production and its function during pregnancy.
2. Describe the principle of the hCG one-step urine device.
3. List the reagents required and the specimen type used with an hCG one-step urine device.
4. List the general steps performed with the hCG one-step urine device.
5. Understand the results interpretation of the hCG one-step urine device.

Shortly after fertilization, the developing placenta secretes a glycoprotein hormone called **human chorionic gonadotropin (hCG)** [1]. hCG has several important functions that play a significant role during the course of pregnancy. For instance, hCG promotes angiogenesis and vasculogenesis to support the fetus with maximum blood supply and nutrients throughout pregnancy [2–8]. Moreover, hCG promotes **progesterone** production, and the production of cytokines such as **macrophage migration inhibitory factor,** which minimize macrophage phagocytosis at the placenta–uterine border, protecting the foreign fetoplacental tissue from destruction [9–11]. Therefore, hCG prevents the rejection of fetoplacental tissue by the maternal immune system. Additionally, it has been reported that hCG stimulates the uterus expansion during the course of pregnancy to fit the fetus size [12, 13]. During healthy pregnancy and as early as 7–10 days post-conception both urine and serum samples show detectable levels of hCG that rapidly continue to increase [14–17]. For this reason, hCG is used as a perfect marker for detecting pregnancy at an early stage. Two types of tests are available to detect pregnancy by measuring hCG, blood, and urine. A blood test, can detect pregnancy earlier than the urine test because of its high sensitivity; however, it has to be performed in clinical laboratories using a sandwich ELISA [18]. Therefore, the blood test is more expensive and requires more time than the hCG one-step pregnancy urine test device, which can be

© Springer International Publishing AG, part of Springer Nature 2018
R. Y. Alhabbab, *Basic Serological Testing*, Techniques in Life Science and Biomedicine for the Non-Expert, https://doi.org/10.1007/978-3-319-77694-1_13

done at home within 2–10 min with high accuracy. An hCG one-step pregnancy urine device can detect hCG at 25 mIU/ml or greater [19].

HCG One-Step Pregnancy Urine Test Device

Principle

Lateral flow chromatographic immunoassay is the method used to qualitatively detect hCG in urine during the early stages of pregnancy [20]. The device contains two windows, the specimen window or well, which contains the sample pad, and the results window. The results window consists of two lines, the control and the test (T) lines [20]. Urine that contains hCG binds to mouse monoclonal anti-hCG conjugated to colloidal gold (gold nanoparticles), which has unique optical and physical properties and produces color when reacting with light, depending on their shape, size, and aggregation state, contained on the conjugate or reagent pad [20]. The complex forms in the reagent or conjugate pad migrate through the membrane strip (usually nitrocellulose or cellulose acetate membrane) and binds to the specific monoclonal anti-hCG antibodies lining the T line, producing color [20]. On the other hand, the control line contains goat anti-mouse antibodies that bind to the mouse monoclonal anti-hCG antibodies of the reagent pad in the presence or absence of hCG (Fig. 13.1) [20]. Therefore, the absence of a colored line at the control line indicates invalid results.

Reagents

Specimens and an hCG one-step pregnancy urine test device.

Steps

1. Bring the urine sample and the test device to room temperature.
2. After removing the test device from its case, add four drops into the sample window or well. This step may vary depending on the manufacturer [20].
3. Read the results after 2–10 min.

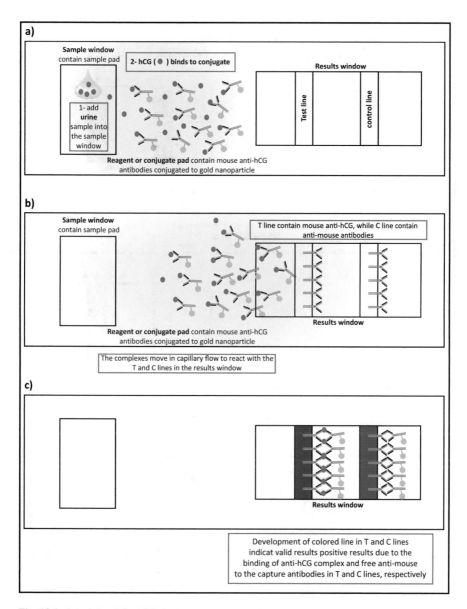

Fig. 13.1 Principle of the hCG one-step pregnancy urine test device

Results Interpretation

For positive results, both T and C lines must produce color to indicate the presence of hCG in the sample at a level equal to or higher than 25 mIU/ml (Fig. 13.2a).

For negative results, only the C line should produce color (Fig. 13.2b).

The results are invalid if the C line does not produce color (Fig. 13.2c).

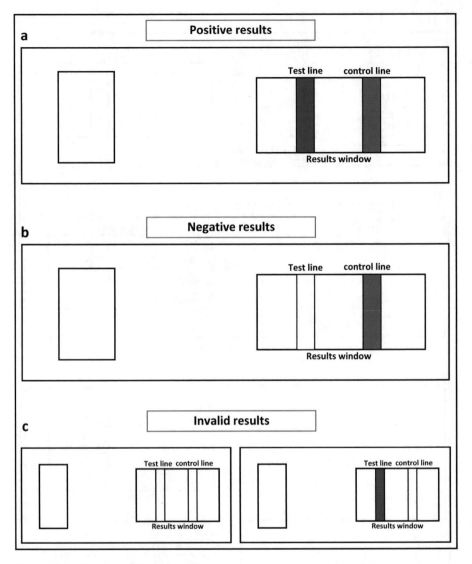

Fig. 13.2 Results interpretation of the hCG one-step pregnancy urine test device

References

1. Ezcurra D, Humaidan P. A review of luteinising hormone and human chorionic gonadotropin when used in assisted reproductive technology. Reprod Biol Endocrinol. 2014;12:95.
2. Berndt S, Blacher S, Perrier d'Hauterive S, Thiry M, Tsampalas M, Cruz A, et al. Chorionic gonadotropin stimulation of angiogenesis and pericyte recruitment. J Clin Endocrinol Metab. 2009;94(11):4567–74.

3. Toth P, Li X, Rao CV, Lincoln SR, Sanfilippo JS, Spinnato JA 2nd, et al. Expression of functional human chorionic gonadotropin/human luteinizing hormone receptor gene in human uterine arteries. J Clin Endocrinol Metab. 1994;79(1):307–15.

4. Lei ZM, Reshef E, Rao V. The expression of human chorionic gonadotropin/luteinizing hormone receptors in human endometrial and myometrial blood vessels. J Clin Endocrinol Metab. 1992;75(2):651–9.

5. Zygmunt M, Herr F, Keller-Schoenwetter S, Kunzi-Rapp K, Munstedt K, Rao CV, et al. Characterization of human chorionic gonadotropin as a novel angiogenic factor. J Clin Endocrinol Metab. 2002;87(11):5290–6.

6. Herr F, Baal N, Reisinger K, Lorenz A, McKinnon T, Preissner KT, et al. HCG in the regulation of placental angiogenesis. Results of an in vitro study. Placenta. 2007;28(Suppl A):S85–93.

7. Zygmunt M, Herr F, Munstedt K, Lang U, Liang OD. Angiogenesis and vasculogenesis in pregnancy. Eur J Obstet Gynecol Reprod Biol. 2003;110(Suppl 1):S10–8.

8. Toth P, Lukacs H, Gimes G, Sebestyen A, Pasztor N, Paulin F, et al. Clinical importance of vascular LH/hCG receptors—a review. Reprod Biol. 2001;1(2):5–11.

9. Akoum A, Metz CN, Morin M. Marked increase in macrophage migration inhibitory factor synthesis and secretion in human endometrial cells in response to human chorionic gonadotropin hormone. J Clin Endocrinol Metab. 2005;90(5):2904–10.

10. Kobayashi S, Nishihira J, Watanabe S, Todo S. Prevention of lethal acute hepatic failure by antimacrophage migration inhibitory factor antibody in mice treated with bacille Calmette-Guerin and lipopolysaccharide. Hepatology. 1999;29(6):1752–9.

11. Wan H, Versnel MA, Cheung WY, Leenen PJ, Khan NA, Benner R, et al. Chorionic gonadotropin can enhance innate immunity by stimulating macrophage function. J Leukoc Biol. 2007;82(4):926–33.

12. Reshef E, Lei ZM, Rao CV, Pridham DD, Chegini N, Luborsky JL. The presence of gonadotropin receptors in nonpregnant human uterus, human placenta, fetal membranes, and decidua. J Clin Endocrinol Metab. 1990;70(2):421–30.

13. Zuo J, Lei ZM, Rao CV. Human myometrial chorionic gonadotropin/luteinizing hormone receptors in preterm and term deliveries. J Clin Endocrinol Metab. 1994;79(3):907–11.

14. Batzer FR. Hormonal evaluation of early pregnancy. Fertil Steril. 1980;34(1):1–13.

15. Catt KJ, Dufau ML, Vaitukaitis JL. Appearance of hCG in pregnancy plasma following the initiation of implantation of the blastocyst. J Clin Endocrinol Metab. 1975;40(3):537–40.

16. Braunstein GD, Rasor J, Danzer H, Adler D, Wade ME. Serum human chorionic gonadotropin levels throughout normal pregnancy. Am J Obstet Gynecol. 1976;126(6):678–81.

17. Lenton EA, Neal LM, Sulaiman R. Plasma concentrations of human chorionic gonadotropin from the time of implantation until the second week of pregnancy. Fertil Steril. 1982;37(6):773–8.

18. BioVision Inc. Chorionic gonadotropin (hCG) (human) ELISA kit. Biovision. Available from: http://www.biovision.com/documentation/datasheets/K7424.pdf. Accessed 20 September 2017.

19. Innovacon. One Step Pregnancy Test Device (Urine). CLIA-waived. Available from: https://www.cliawaived.com/web/items/pdf/FHC102_Innovacon_hcG_Pregnancy_Device~1671file1.pdf. Accessed 20 September 2017.

20. CLIAwaived Inc. Pregnancy Urine Test (Cassette). CLIA-waived. Available from: https://www.cliawaived.com/web/items/pdf/CLIA_02_2478_25_hCG_Pregnancy_Cassette~2242file2.pdf. Accessed 20 September 2017.

Study Questions

1. **Human chronic gonadotropin (hCG) is:**

   (a) An enzyme.
   (b) **Hormone**.
   (c) Carbohydrate.
   (d) Complement protein.

2. **hCG produced during:**

   (a) **Pregnancy**.
   (b) Autoimmune diseases.
   (c) Cancer.
   (d) Post-transplant.

3. **hCG functions include:**

   (a) Helping to support the fetus during pregnancy with nutrients and blood supply.
   (b) Promoting cytokine production.
   (c) Promoting progesterone production
   (d) **All the above**.

4. **hCG can be detected in both urine and blood at:**

   (a) A month after conception.
   (b) **A week post-conception**.
   (c) Three months post-conception.
   (d) None of the above.

5. **hCG can be detected in:**

   (a) **Urine and blood**.
   (b) Vaginal swab.
   (c) Saliva.
   (d) None of the above.

6. **An hCG one-step pregnancy urine device can detect hCG at:**

   (a) **25 mIU/ml or greater**.
   (b) 15 mIU/ml.
   (c) 10 mIU/ml.
   (d) 5 mIU/ml.

7. **The principle of the hCG one-step pregnancy urine device is:**

   (a) ELISA.
   (b) PCR.
   (c) **Chromatography**.
   (d) Latex agglutination.

8. **A conjugate pad of hCG one-step pregnancy urine device contains:**

   (a) Anti-hCG conjugated to an enzyme.
   (b) **Anti-hCG conjugated to gold nanoparticles.**
   (c) Anti-hCG conjugated to a protein.
   (d) Anti-hCG conjugated to a biotin.

9. **A C line on the results window of the hCG one-step pregnancy urine device contains:**

   (a) Anti-hCG antibodies.
   (b) **Anti-mouse antibodies.**
   (c) Anti-goat antibodies.
   (d) None of the above.

10. **The result of the hCG one-step pregnancy urine device is:**

    (a) Positive.
    (b) Negative.
    (c) **Invalid.**
    (d) None of the above.

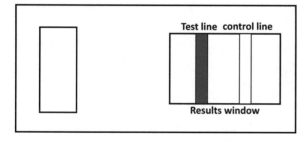

Chapter 14
Radial Immunodiffusion (RID)

Learning Objectives
By the end of this chapter the reader should be able to:

1. Describe the RID principle.
2. List the reagents required and the specimen type used in RID.
3. List the general steps performed in RID.
4. Understand the results interpretation of RID.

Radial immunodiffusion (RID) assay is a quantitative method used in many clinical laboratories to determine the concentration of specific antigens or antibody classes (IgG, IgA, and IgM) in patient serum.

Radial Immunodiffusion (RID) Assay

Principle

This quantitative method depends on the formation of antigen-antibodies complexes in **agarose gel**. Sera that contain antibodies or antigens diffuse through the agarose gel, which contains antibodies specific to the target antigen or antibodies in the patient serum [1, 2]. As antigens or antibodies in patient serum diffuse via the gel, they form complexes with the specific antibodies in the gel radically in all directions. Antigen–antibody complexes precipitate, forming a ring (**precipitin ring**) around the sample well [1, 2]. The ring size is the equivalence point where the antigens or antibodies concentration in the sample and antibodies in the agarose gel are equally proportioned. The concentration of antigens or antibodies is proportional to the diameter of the precipitin ring (Fig. 14.1) [1, 2].

The most common RID in serology is one that measures IgG, IgA, and IgM concentrations; therefore, it is the test described in this chapter.

© Springer International Publishing AG, part of Springer Nature 2018   105
R. Y. Alhabbab, *Basic Serological Testing*, Techniques in Life Science and
Biomedicine for the Non-Expert, https://doi.org/10.1007/978-3-319-77694-1_14

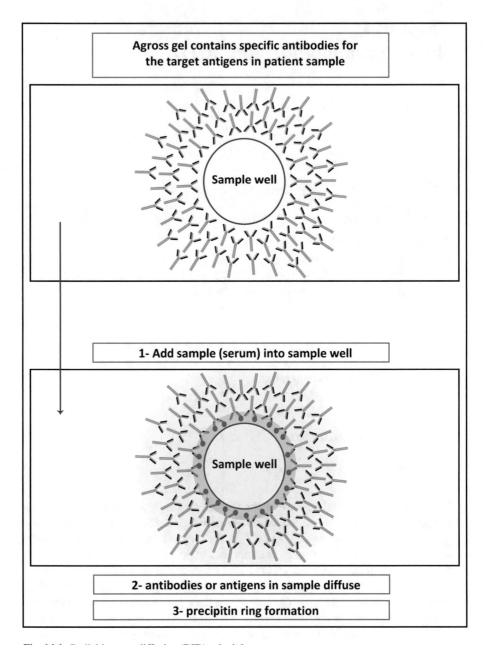

Fig. 14.1 Radial immunodiffusion (RID) principle

Reagents

1. An RID plate: usually ready to use agarose gel containing antibodies specific to IgG, IgA or IgM in a plate. The plate contains a number of wells depending on the manufacturer [2].
2. Calibrators or standards: contain known concentrations of IgG, IgA, and IgM.
3. Control serum: one vial of a known concentration for IgG, IgA, and IgM.

Steps

1. Bring the RID plate, samples, control, and calibrators to room temperature.
2. Add 5–10 µl from samples, control, and calibrators to the appropriate well [2].
3. Cover with the plate lid and incubate at room temperature in a flat position as follows:

   72 h for IgA and IgG [2].
   96 h for IgM [2].

   Note: During incubation, the plate should not be allowed to dry out. Therefore, it should be incubated in a moist box.

Results Interpretation

1. After incubation, measure the diameter of the precipitin ring of the calibrators, control and samples.
2. Plot the diameter size of the precipitin ring of the calibrators onto a graph, as shown in Fig. 14.2a [1, 2].
3. To determine the immunoglobulin concentration in patient serum using the calibration curve, draw a horizontal line out of the *y*-axis from the diameter value of the precipitin ring to reach the calibration curve, as shown in Fig. 14.2b [1, 2].
4. From the point of intersection, drop a second vertical line to the *x*-axis, as illustrated in Fig. 14.2c [1, 2].
5. Record the antibody concentrations.

However, some kits do not require a calibration curve because they provide an RID reference table, which encloses the concentrations of each diameter that can possibly be obtained from the gel.

Fig. 14.2 Results
interpretation of RID

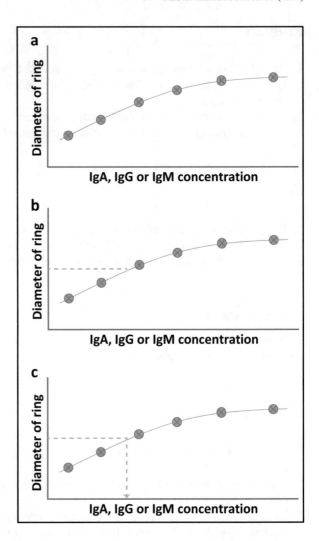

References

1. HiMedical Laboratories. Hiper Radial Immunodiffusion Teaching Kit. himediallabs. Available from: http://himedialabs.com/TD/HTI004.pdf. Accessed 21 September 2017.
2. Human IgG, IgA & IgM 'NL' Bindarid Radial Immunodiffusion Kits. cosmobio. 2005. Available from: http://search.cosmobio.co.jp/cosmo_search_p/search_gate2/docs/BDS_/ RN0103.20070813.pdf. Accessed 21 September 2017.

Study Questions

1. **The RID method depends on:**

   (a) **Precipitation of antigens–antibodies complexes**.
   (b) Agglutination of latex particles.
   (c) Agglutination of RBCs.
   (d) None of the above.

2. **RID requires:**

   (a) Gel electrophoresis.
   (b) **Agarose gel**.
   (c) Polyacrylamide gel.
   (d) Cellulose acetate membrane.

3. **The antigen concentration in RID is:**

   (a) **Proportional to the diameter of the precipitin ring**.
   (b) Double the diameter of the precipitin ring.
   (c) Half the diameter of the precipitin ring.
   (d) None of the above.

4. **The incubation time required for IgM measured by RID is:**

   (a) 12 h.
   (b) 24 h.
   (c) 72 h.
   (d) **96 h**.

5. **RID plates should be:**

   (a) Dried out.
   (b) **Kept in a moist environment**.
   (c) Heated before results measurement.
   (d) Incubated at 4 °C.

6. **RID results measurements require:**

   (a) **A calibration curve**.
   (b) A plate reader.
   (c) A microscope.
   (d) A rotator.

Chapter 15
Immunofixation Electrophoresis (IFE)

Learning Objectives
By the end of this chapter the reader should be able to:

1. Describe the principle of IFE.
2. List the reagents required and the specimen type used in IFE.
3. List the general steps performed in IFE.
4. Understand the results interpretation for IFE.

Immunofixation electrophoresis (IFE) is the gold standard technique in clinical immunology laboratories to quantify and identify **M protein**, which is also called M-band or paraprotein [1]. The quantity and isotype of M protein are important in the diagnosis and follow-up of **monoclonal gammopathies (MG)** [1]. MG severity can be as benign as monoclonal gammopathy of undetermined significance (MGUS) or as severe as light chain amyloidosis (AL) [1]. M protein of less than 3 g/dl together with clonal plasma cells of less than 10% in bone marrow with no end organ damage is considered to indicate MGUS [2]. MGUS may progress over the years into a more severe form of MG, such as multiple myeloma, AL, Waldenstrom macroglobulinemia or lymphoma [2]. Risk of progression is determined by the size and type of serum M protein and by the number of plasma cells in the bone marrow, along with the ratio of the serum free light chain (FLC) [2]. Serum protein electrophoresis, serum IFE, and FLC are the three methods used in clinical immunology laboratories to screen for M protein in myeloma patients or related disorders [2, 3]. However, M protein is detected preferably by agarose gel electrophoresis and the presence of localized protein or band on the agarose gel must be confirmed by IFE, which also identifies the isotype of M protein (heavy and light chains).

© Springer International Publishing AG, part of Springer Nature 2018
R. Y. Alhabbab, *Basic Serological Testing*, Techniques in Life Science and
Biomedicine for the Non-Expert, https://doi.org/10.1007/978-3-319-77694-1_15

Immunofixation Electrophoresis

Principle

Agarose Gel Electrophoresis

The separation of proteins by agarose gel electrophoresis depends on several factors such as the size, charge, and shape of the tested molecules, and the gel concentration [4]. Therefore, the protein molecules are separated according to their molecular weight, where smaller and more compact molecules move faster than larger and more elongated molecules in an electrically charged field [4]. In addition, negatively charged molecules move faster toward the positive anode pole. Moreover, using gel with a low agarose concentration, the protein travels faster than in a gel with a high agarose concentration [4].

IFE

The principle of IFE includes the addition of anti-sera such as anti-IgG, anti-IgA, anti-IgM, anti-α-κ, and anti-α-λ chain antibodies to the agarose gel or cellulose acetate membrane after electrophoresis, and at antigen–antibodies equivalence, or in moderate antibody excess, the antibodies and antigens develop large precipitates in the gel or cellulose acetate membrane [5]. After washing the gel or the membrane, free proteins and unbound antibodies are washed out, leaving the large and insoluble immunoprecipitates in the gel or membrane pores [5]. Staining the immunoprecipitates directly identifies the isotype of the M protein (Fig. 15.1).

Reagents

Agarose Gel Requirements and Preparation

1. Large beaker.
2. Tris-barbital buffer (TBA).
3. Agarose.
4. Microwave.
5. Gel plate.
6. Combs.
7. Gel box.
8. Ladder: consists of standard proteins to identify the approximate size of the molecules running through the gel.
9. Loading dye: contains a dye that enables the protein movement in the gel to be visualized, and sucrose or glycerol to make the sample denser than the running buffer and prevent it from floating.
10. Electrical field.

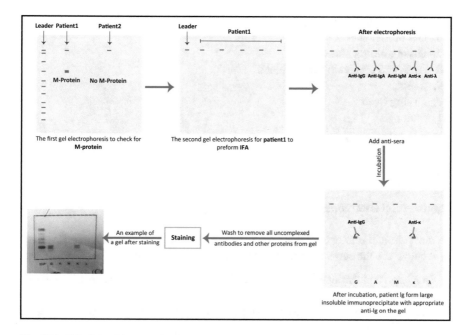

Fig. 15.1 Principle of immunofixation electrophoresis (IFE)

Cellulose Acetate (Cellogel) Membrane Electrophoresis

1. TBA.
2. Cellogel strips.
3. Electrophoresis chamber.
4. Filter paper.
5. Strip bridges.
6. Plastic clips.
7. Sample holder.
8. Destaining solution.
9. Cleaning solution.
10. Mylar film or glass slide.
11. Glass rod.
12. Drying oven.
13. Densitometry.

IFE

1. Labeled agarose gel or cellogel strips.
2. Gel blotter strips.
3. Sample applicator or template.
4. Pipette.

5. Electrophoresis chamber.
6. Gel blotter sheets.
7. Drying blotter sheets.
8. Anti-sera applicator or template.
9. Saline.
10. Drying oven.
11. Stain.

Steps

Agarose Gel Electrophoresis

In most clinical immune laboratories ready-to-use agarose gel is utilized. However, below are the steps required to prepare in-house agarose gel.

1. In a large beaker put 80 ml of TBA and 0.8 g of agarose to prepare 0.8% agarose gel.
2. Place the beaker in a microwave until boiling. At boiling point, pull the beaker out and swirl.
3. Repeat heating and swirl until the agarose dissolves completely in the TBA.
4. Seal the gel plate to prevent the gel from leaking and put combs into the gel plate, then pour the prepared agarose gel into the plate.
5. After a while, the gel will solidify, remove the seal and the combs from the gel plate and put the plate into the gel box.
6. Pour 1× TBA into the gel box (cover the gel).
7. Mix the ladder and the patient samples with the loading buffer and then load them into the gel wells.
8. Cover the box and generate an electrical field by applying a current that allows the movement of the proteins through the gel.
9. Stain the gel with acid violet stain to visualize the M protein.

Cellulose Acetate (Cellogel) Membrane Electrophoresis

1. Put about 100 ml of TBA buffer into a container, then immerse the cellogel strips in the buffer, and place the buffer container on a shaker for 10 min.
2. Fill up the electrophoresis chamber completely with TBA buffer, and ensure that both compartments are filled equally.
3. Apply 30 μl of samples into the semimicro drop holder (or sample holder).
4. Gently dry cellogel strips by placing them between two filter paper sheets, then place the strip bridges (penetrable surface up), and hold the strip on the strip bridge by the plastic chips from both sides.
5. Place the strip bridge immediately into the electrophoresis chamber.

6. Put dH$_2$O into the base of the sample holder, and prime the applicator by depressing the tips of the applicator on the first row of the semimicro drop holder or sample holder and apply the load onto the filter paper.
7. Load the applicator again from the sample on the first row and apply it to the strip bridge (on the negative pole).
8. Cover the electrophoresis chamber and apply the current.
9. After the electrophoresis has been done, remove the cellogel strips from the strip bridge and immerse it in a container containing about 100 ml of Ponceau S solution for 5 min on a shaker.
10. Destain the cellogel strips in a container containing destaining solution until the background of the cellogel strip returns to white (on shaker).
11. Place the destained strip into a container containing cleaning solution for 30 min.
12. Put the strip on Mylar film or a glass slide and using a glass rod remove all the excess solution.
13. Dry the strips by putting them in a drying oven at 70–80 °C for 10 min.
14. After cooling the strips to room temperature, the film is ready for **densitometry** (an optical system to generate an electropherogram, a diagram of separated bands).

IFE

1. After running the electrophoresis for patients with M protein on a new labeled agarose gel or cellogel membrane, put the anti-sera template on the gel and ensure that there are no air bubbles; then, apply the appropriate anti-sera and incubate for about 20 min at 15–25 °C.
2. After incubation and discarding the anti-sera template, dry the gel by applying a blotter sheet and a drying blotter sheet for 5 min under pressure.
3. Wash the film in saline for 10 min, and dry it as described above.
4. Repeat steps 2 and 3 twice.
5. Stain the film and evaluate the results.

Results Interpretation

An electropherogram is generated by using an optical system called a densitometer [6]. An electropherogram is created after staining the electrophoresis gel that has passed via the densitometer system. Serum proteins are divided into five classes according to their electrical charge, including albumin, alpha1, alpha2, beta, and gamma [6]. Figure 15.2 shows an example of protein-separated bands from serum samples of normal and M protein containing one.

The presence of M protein in patient serum requires identifying the isotypes of the M protein using IFE (Fig. 15.3).

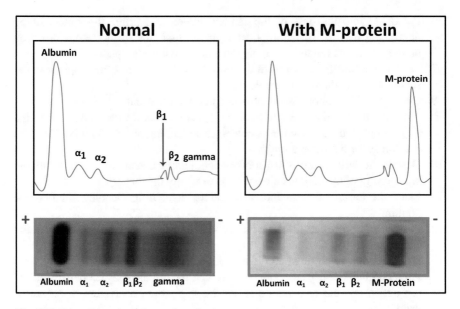

Fig. 15.2   M protein on gel electrophoresis

Fig. 15.3   Results of IFE

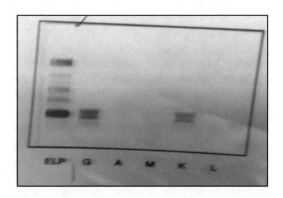

Figure 15.3 illustrates an example of IFE results showing an M protein that is mainly IgG with a κ light chain.

References

1. Tate J, Mollee P, Johnson R. Monoclonal gammopathies – clinical and laboratory issues. Clin Biochem Rev. 2009;30(3):89–91.
2. Kyle RA, Rajkumar SV. Management of monoclonal gammopathy of undetermined significance (MGUS) and smoldering multiple myeloma (SMM). Oncology (Williston Park). 2011;25(7):578–86.

3. Katzmann JA, Dispenzieri A, Kyle RA, Snyder MR, Plevak MF, Larson DR, et al. Elimination of the need for urine studies in the screening algorithm for monoclonal gammopathies by using serum immunofixation and free light chain assays. Mayo Clin Proc. 2006;81(12):1575–8.
4. Yılmaz M, Ozic C, Gok I. Principles of nucleic acid separation by agarose gel electrophoresis, gel electrophoresis – principles and basics. In Magdeldin S (Ed.), InTech. https://doi.org/10.5772/38654. 2012. Available from: https://www.intechopen.com/books/gel-electrophoresis-principles-and-basics/principles-of-nucleic-acid-separation-by-agarose-gel-electrophoresis. Accessed 30 September 2017.
5. Csako G. Immunofixation electrophoresis for identification of proteins and specific antibodies. Methods Mol Biol. 2012;869:147–71.
6. Bansal F, Bhagat P, Srinivasan VK, Chhabra S, Gupta P. Immunoglobulin A gammopathy on serum electrophoresis: a diagnostic conundrum. Indian J Pathol Microbiol. 2016;59(1):134–6.

Study Questions

1. **IFE is commonly used in serology to:**

   (a) **Identify M proteins.**
   (b) Identify HBV.
   (c) Measure antibodies.
   (d) Measure complements.

2. **The M protein isotype is important in patients with:**

   (a) HBV
   (b) **Monoclonal gammopathies.**
   (c) Hemolytic anemia
   (d) Systemic lupus erythematosus.

3. **Screening for M protein is usually by:**

   (a) **Electrophoresis.**
   (b) Radial immunodiffusion.
   (c) IFE
   (d) All the above.

4. **Protein separation by agarose gel electrophoresis depends on:**

   (a) The size of the proteins.
   (b) The shape of the proteins.
   (c) The charge of the proteins.
   (d) **All the above.**

5. **A high concentration of agarose in a gel leads to:**

   (a) Fast protein separation.
   (b) **Slow protein separation.**
   (c) None of the above.

6. **IFE utilizes:**

   (a) Anti-IgG antibodies.
   (b) Anti-IgM antibodies.
   (c) Anti-IgA antibodies.
   (d) **All the above**.

7. **Function/s of loading dye in agarose electrophoresis is/are:**

   (a) Complement activation.
   (b) **Making the sample denser**.
   (c) Identifying the size of the protein bands.
   (d) Identifying the shape of the proteins.

Chapter 16
Immunofluorescence (IF) Assay

Learning Objectives
By the end of this chapter the reader should be able to:

1. Describe the principles of each IF type.
2. List the reagents required and the specimen type used in IF.
3. List the general steps performed in IF.
4. Understand results interpretation of IF.

Immunofluorescence (IF) is a histochemical laboratory staining technique that relies on antibodies–antigens interactions in tissue or body fluids [1, 2]. **IF** is broadly used in clinical immunology laboratories to help in the diagnosis of autoimmune diseases and in patients' treatment and monitoring.

Immunofluorescence (IF) Assay

Principle

The IF test is available in four basic types, **direct IF**, **indirect IF** (the most commonly used in the clinical immunology laboratory), **indirect IF complement fixation**, and **double IF**.

Direct IF

Direct IF is a technique where fluorescently labeled antibody specific to the target antigen is used in a patient tissue or cell [2]. It is a one-step procedure that uses only one primary conjugated antibody [2] (Fig. 16.1).

© Springer International Publishing AG, part of Springer Nature 2018   119
R. Y. Alhabbab, *Basic Serological Testing*, Techniques in Life Science and
Biomedicine for the Non-Expert, https://doi.org/10.1007/978-3-319-77694-1_16

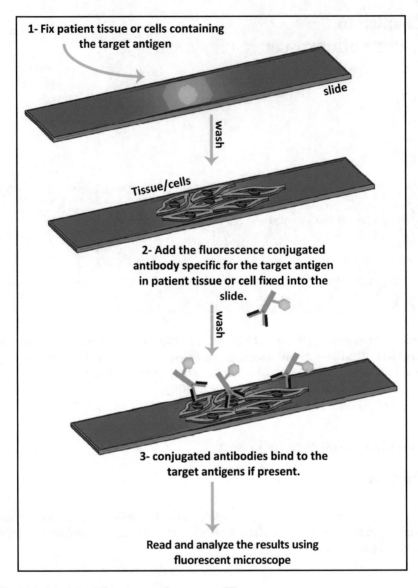

Fig. 16.1 Principle of direct immunofluorescence (IF)

Indirect IF

Indirect IF is usually used to detect specific patient antibodies. It is performed in two steps, the first step using unlabeled antibodies (patient antibodies), and the second step requires using secondary antibodies that are specific to the Fc region and labeled with fluorescence (Fig. 16.2) [1, 3, 4].

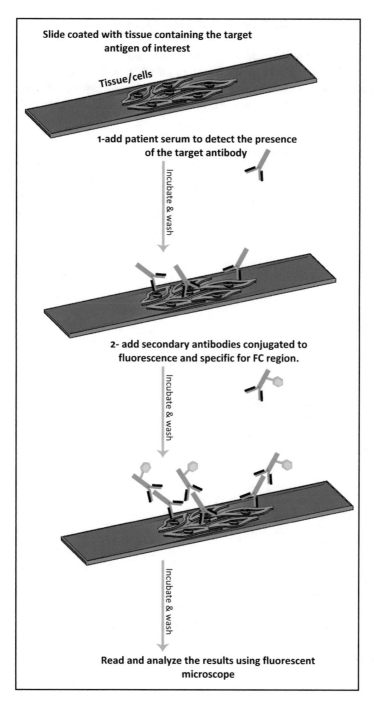

Fig. 16.2 Principle of indirect IF

Indirect Immunofluorescence Complement Fixation

Indirect immunofluorescence complement fixation (IF-CF) is more sensitive than indirect IF because it uses an amplification principle [1, 3, 4]. Here, the generation of antigen–antibody complexes activates the complement system to release C3 molecules that are detected by anti-C3 conjugated to fluorochrome (Fig. 16.3) [1–3].

Double Immunofluorescence

Double immunofluorescence (DIF) allows the detection of two different antibodies on cells by using two specific antibodies for the target antigens. Each is labeled with a different fluorochrome such as FITC (fluorescein) and rhodamine [1]. This technique can be used with direct and indirect IF methods [1].

Reagents

Direct IF

1. Specimen (skin or mucosal biopsy).
2. Cryostat.
3. Glass slide.
4. Phosphate-buffered saline (PBS).
5. Moist chamber.
6. Conjugated antibody specific to the antigen of interest.
7. Buffered glycerin.
8. Fluorescent microscope.

Indirect IF

1. Substrate section.
2. Glass slide.
3. Patient sample (serum).
4. Moist chamber.
5. PBS.
6. FITC-conjugated secondary antibodies specific for Fc region.
7. Glycerin.
8. Fluorescent microscope.

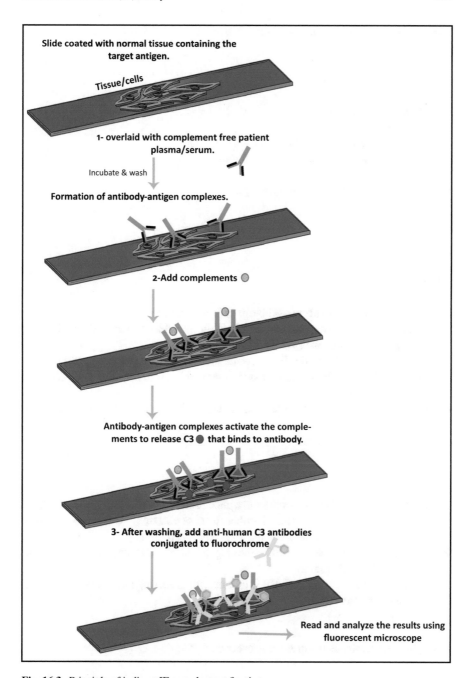

Fig. 16.3 Principle of indirect IF complement fixation

Complement Indirect Immunofluorescence

1. Tissue substrate.
2. Glass slide.
3. PBS.
4. Patient sample (serum).
5. Heating source.
6. Complement source such as fresh human serum.
7. FITC-conjugated anti-human C3 antibodies.
8. Glycerin.
9. Cover slip and fluorescent microscope.

Steps

Direct IF

1. Patient sample (skin or mucosal biopsy) is snap frozen.
2. About 4–6µl of the snap-frozen sample is sectioned using a cryostat and placed on a glass slide, and air-dried for 15 min [1].
3. After washing by PBS, the FITC-conjugated antibodies that are specific to the antigens of interest in the patient sample are added into the slide and incubated in a moist chamber.
4. Wash, mount with glycerin, place on the cover slip, and examine under the fluorescent microscope.

Indirect IF

1. After placing the substrate section on a glass slide, add the serially diluted patient serum, and incubate in a moist chamber for about 30 min. Positive and negative control sera must be used to test the antibody reactivity [1].
2. Wash with PBS, and add the FITC-conjugated antibodies that are specific to the human antibody Fc region.
3. Wash for at least 10 min with PBS, mount with glycerin, and examine under the fluorescent microscope.

Complement Indirect Immunofluorescence

1. After placing the substrate section on a glass slide, add the patient serum or plasma that was heated at 56 °C for 30 min to destroy all complement without affecting the antigens or antibodies present in the serum [1].

2. Add the complement source. The complement system is activated by the antibodies that are bound to the antigen on the slide, releasing numerous C3 molecules that bind to the antigen–antibody complexes [1].
3. After washing, add the FITC-conjugated antibodies specific to human C3, then wash, mount, and examine under the fluorescent microscope [1].

Results Interpretation

1. If no fluorescence is detected under the fluorescent microscope, it is a negative sample.
2. According to the binding pattern of the anti-nuclear antibodies and the intensity of the fluorescence (1^+, 2^+, 3^+ or 4^+), the autoimmune disease can be determined in correlation with the ELISA results for double-stranded DNA, single-stranded DNA, and histone [5, 6].

References

1. Mohan KH, Pai S, Rao R, Sripathi H, Prabhu S. Techniques of immunofluorescence and their significance. Indian J Dermatol Venereol Leprol. 2008;74(4):415–9.
2. Betterle C, Zanchetta R. The immunofluorescence techniques in the diagnosis of endocrine autoimmune diseases. Auto Immun Highlights. 2012;3(2):67–78.
3. Huilgol SC, Bhogal BS, Black MM. Immunofluorescence of the immunobullous disorders: Part two: The clinical disorders. Indian J Dermatol Venereol Leprol. 1995;61(5):255–64.
4. Vassileva S. Immunofluorescence in dermatology. Int J Dermatol. 1993;32(3):153–61.
5. Kern P, Kron M, Hiesche K. Measurement of antinuclear antibodies: assessment of different test systems. Clin Diagn Lab Immunol. 2000;7(1):72–8.
6. Mengeloglu Z, Tas T, Kocoglu E, Aktas G, Karabork S. Determination of anti-nuclear antibody pattern distribution and clinical relationship. Pak J Med Sci. 2014;30(2):380–3.

Study Questions

1. **IF is used in the immune laboratory to:**

   (a) Detect pregnancy.
   (b) **Diagnose autoimmune disorder**.
   (c) Cross-match tissue.
   (d) Detect cancer.

2. **IF types include:**

   (a) Direct
   (b) Indirect.

(c) IF-CF.

(d) **All the above**.

3. **Patient samples that are used with direct IF are:**

(a) Whole blood.

(b) Serum.

(c) Plasma.

(d) **Tissue or cells**.

4. **Indirect IF requires:**

(a) Primary antibodies.

(b) **Primary and secondary antibodies**.

(c) Complement.

(d) None of the above.

5. **Complement activation in IF-CF depends on:**

(a) **The presence of antigen–antibody complexes**.

(b) The presence of RBCs.

(c) The presence of free antibodies.

(d) None of the above.

6. **Double immunofluorescence is characterized by:**

(a) **The ability to detect two different antibodies in a patient sample**.

(b) The ability to kill pathogens.

(c) The ability to detect cytokines.

(d) The ability to detect and activate complements.

7. **Direct IF requires:**

(a) **A cryostat**.

(b) A rotator.

(c) A water bath.

(d) A light microscope.

Glossary

Acute phase proteins play a key role in the early phase response to infection and include several cytokines such as IL-6, IL1, TNF, and IFN in addition to C-reactive proteins.

Adaptive immunity is a specific immune response mainly carried out by lymphocytes and has the ability to develop immunological memory.

Affinity is the binding constant measurement of a single antigen binding site with its epitope.

Agarose gel electrophoresis is an electrophoresis method that uses agarose, which consists of polysaccharide polymer. Agarose gel forms linear polymers consisting of repeating units to separate large protein molecules.

Agglutination requires antibodies to aggregate certain antigens.

Alternative complement pathway is the mechanism that directly activates the complement system via the activation of C3 and C3b deposition on cell surface.

Antibodies are serum proteins produced by plasma cells in response to immunogens and binds specifically to antigens.

Antibody Fc region is the region of an antibody that contains the constant domain.

Antibody Fab region is the region of an antibody that contains two specific antigen-binding sites with the same specificity.

Anti-citrullinated protein antibodies (ACPAs) are autoantibodies against peptides/protein epitopes that are citrullinated and found in RA especially during the early stages of the disease.

Antigen-presenting cells (APCs) express MHC class II molecules, which present peptides from processed phagocytosed antigens to T cells.

Antigens are any foreign molecules that specifically bind to lymphocytes or antibodies.

Anti-streptolysin O (ASO/ASL) is an antibody produced by host plasma cells against the endotoxins (streptolysin O) that are produced by group A streptococcus. This antibody is usually used in serology to detect previous and current infections.

© Springer International Publishing AG, part of Springer Nature 2018
R. Y. Alhabbab, *Basic Serological Testing*, Techniques in Life Science and
Biomedicine for the Non-Expert, https://doi.org/10.1007/978-3-319-77694-1

Autoantibodies are antibodies that cause damage to tissue and cells because they are produced to attack self-antigens.

Autoimmune disorders are the failure of the immune system to identify self-antigens as non-foreign and start attacking the body tissue, producing several immunological components. Most importantly, antibodies specific to such tissue are called autoantibodies.

Avidity is the sum of several affinities.

B cell receptors (BCRs) are expressed at the membrane surface of B cells; BCRs are specific and consist of transmembrane immunoglobulin bound non-covalently to invariant Igα and Igβ chains.

B cells are lymphocytes that develop and mature in the bone marrow, and they are the precursors of the cells that produce antibodies (plasma cells).

Brucella is a zoonotic intracellular bacterial infection. The most pathogenic *Brucella* species to humans are *B. melitensis*, *B. suis*, *B. abortus*, and *B. canis*.

C1q is a component of C1, and the first protein involved in the classical complement pathway.

C3 is the first and the fourth component of the alternative and the classical complement pathways respectively.

CD8 T cells (cytotoxic T cells) is a T cell population that expresses CD8 and interacts with MHC class I expressed on virally infected and tumor cells, and kills these cells, mainly by producing cytoplasmic granules, which results in target cell apoptosis.

Chronic inflammation is an inflammatory response that occurs over a prolonged period.

Classical complement pathway is the mechanism that activates the complement system via antigen–antibody complexes.

Clonal deletion is the elimination of specific lymphocytes cloned following their activation with either foreign or self-antigens.

Clonal selection theory is the concept that the specificity and diversity of the immune responses are the consequences of the selection of specific reactive clones from a large repertoire of existing lymphocytes by antigens.

Clonal expansion is the process that results in an increase in the number of specific lymphocytes.

Competitive ELISA uses two antigens, one is labeled with biotin and the second is the patient antigen competing for the same antibodies.

Complement system is a group of proteins that may be cell-associated and serum proteins and involved in the immune responses against pathogens, either indirectly by recognizing antibody–antigen complexes (classical pathway) or directly by identifying the foreign substance (alternative and lectin pathway).

Complement fixation test measures complement fixation to antibody–antigen complexes and uses sheep red blood cells (sRBCs) as an indicator system.

C-reactive proteins (CRPs) are serum proteins released as a result of inflammation that stimulate the cells of the liver (hepatocytes) to produce them during the acute phase response.

Cytokines produced by almost all cells and are soluble molecules that have several effects on other cells.

Cytotoxic cells include all the immune cells that are capable of killing other cells, such as NK and CD8$^+$ T cells.

Densitometry is a technique that measures the optical density in materials sensitive to light.

Direct agglutination is the direct agglutination of pathogens with its specific antibodies.

Direct ELISA uses one antibody specific to the target antigen and labeled with enzyme; therefore, it is the fastest type of ELISA, but has the lowest level of sensitivity.

Direct hemagglutination is the direct agglutination of pathogens with RBCs.

Double diffusion is the diffusion of two particles, antigens and antibodies, in agar medium to form precipitin at their equivalent point.

Electrophoresis is a method used to separate proteins according to their size, charge, and shape.

Endosome–lysosome mechanism is the degradation of both extracellularly and intracellularly derived proteins into peptides by phagocytic cells containing proteolytic enzymes (lysosome and endosome).

Epitope also called antigenic determinant. Epitopes are specific regions of an antigen that are recognizable by antibodies or TCR.

Equivalence is the point where antigen–antibody interaction is optimal (maximum precipitation).

Fc receptors are expressed by different types of cells and have high and specific affinity to the Fc region of the antibody.

Freeze drying/lymphilizing is a process used to preserve materials by dehydration.

Gel diffusion is a process by which antibodies and antigens diffuse in gel medium to form precipitin.

Glomerulonephritis is a glomerular injury due to deposits of immunoglobulin and complement components in the glomeruli.

Granulocytes see polymorphonuclear cells (PMNs).

Hemolysin is a substance that could be protein or lipid and results in the destruction of the cell membrane of blood cells.

Hemagglutination is the agglutination of a particular antigen by RBCs coated with antibodies.

High sensitivity CRPs (hs-CRPs) are used in serology laboratories to detect CRP and as a cardiovascular disease risk prediction factor.

Homeostasis is the state of immunological balance during regular physiological condition, and the state that the immune system aims to restore after any immunological responses.

Human chorionic gonadotropin (hCG) is a glycoprotein hormone that is secreted by the placenta during the early stages of pregnancy; therefore, it is used in clinical laboratories as a pregnancy indicator.

Humoral responses are the immune responses that involve antibodies.

IgA is mainly produced by the plasma cells of the mucosa-associated lymphoid tissue. IgA is characterized by its α heavy chain.

IgD is expressed on naïve B cells together with IgM and may act as a co-receptor, which binds to IgD receptors on T cells. IgD is characterized by its δ heavy chain.

IgE is mainly associated with allergies and is characterized by its ε heavy chain.

IgG is the only antibody class that can pass through the placenta, and is the highest found in the plasma. IgG is characterized by its γ heavy chain.

IgM is expressed on the B cell surface, and it is the first secreted antibody class following B cell activation. IgM is characterized by its μ heavy chain.

Immunofluorescence (IF) is a method that uses a fluorescent microscope to detect the interaction between fluorescent-labeled conjugates and their target antigens.

Immunogens are molecules that can initiate immune responses.

Immunological memory develops following exposure to a pathogen for the first time that leads to the development of memory cells that can recognize the same pathogen more effectively and rapidly than the first interaction.

Indirect agglutination is the indirect agglutination of a particular antigen with particles coated with specific antibodies for that antigen and vice versa.

Indirect ELISA uses two antibodies: one specific to the target antigen and the second is specific to the first antibody Fc region.

Indirect hemagglutination is the indirect agglutination of antigen coating RBCs by its specific antibodies.

Innate immunity is the first line of defense. It is antigen non-specific, does not develop memory to foreign antigens, and includes several immunological elements and cells such as phagocytic cells and complements.

Interferons (IFNs) consist of several proteins that function as antiviral proteins and can enhance the immune responses.

Ion exchange chromatography is a chromatography technique that separates ions and polar molecules depending on their ion exchange in the solution.

Lateral flow chromatographic immunoassay is a nitrocellulose membrane-based test device that usually contains a sample pad, a conjugate pad that contains anti-sera antibodies for the target antigen in the patient sample, and a result window containing test and control lines.

Lectin complement pathway is the mechanism that activates the complement system by recognizing and binding C2 and C4 to mannan moieties on the pathogen surface.

Lipopolysaccharides (LPS) are molecules expressed on the cell wall of Gram-negative bacteria, also called endotoxins.

Macrophage migration inhibitory factor is a cytokine produced by a variety of cells and plays a pro-inflammatory role in many diseases. It plays a regulatory role in pregnancy.

Macroscopic is used to describe a test result that can be interpreted visually, without the need for a microscope.

Major histocompatibility complex (MHC) is expressed by a variety of cells, is mainly involved in T cell activation, and consists of MHC class I and class II.

Malta fever (Mediterranean) is a bacterial infection caused by *B. melitensis*, called Malta or Mediterranean owing to the very common spread of the disease in these areas.

Membrane attack complex (MAC) is the end result of the activation cascade of the complement components and damages the attacked cells by forming pores on their surface.

Monoclonal gammopathies (MGs) comprise a group of disorders mainly associated with an abnormal immunoglobulin protein called M-protein.

Mononucleosis is a viral infection caused by Epstein–Barr virus.

M-protein is a protein associated with an abnormal immunoglobulin fragment.

Natural killer (NK) cells are lymphocyte-like large granular cells that play a key role in killing virally infected and tumor cells, and do not require previous exposure to antigens.

Non-treponemal test includes RPR and VDRL tests, and is used in clinical laboratories to screen for syphilis. However, it can cross-react with several diseases because it is not specific for syphilis, causing bacteria; therefore, positive results must be confirmed by a treponemal test.

Opsonization is a process that enhances and facilitates phagocytosis by phagocytic cells by coating the target molecules by antibodies or complement components (opsonin).

Pathogen-associated molecular patterns (PAMPs) comprise a group of molecules that have a conserved molecular structure, and are recognized by specialized receptors expressed by cells of the immune system known as PRRs.

Pattern recognition receptors (PRRs) comprise a group of receptors expressed by almost all cells of the immune system, and recognize any non-self-molecules or damaged tissues, subsequently activating the immune system.

Phagocytic cells include several cells such as macrophages, neutrophils, and DCs. The main function of these cells is to engulf any foreign molecules or damaged cells in a process known as phagocytosis.

Plasma cells are responsible for producing antibodies and are differentiated from B cells.

Platelet cells are produced from the bone marrow and play a major role in the formation of blood clots.

Polymorphonuclear (PMN) cells are leukocytes with a multi-lobed nucleolus and include three major cell types: basophils, eosinophils, and neutrophils.

Precipitation requires the formation of insoluble antigen–antibody complexes as a result of mixing soluble antigens and antibodies.

Precipitin ring is a technique for estimating antibody concentration.

Progesterone is a steroid hormone that is secreted by the corpus luteum to prepare the uterus for pregnancy.

Radioimmunoassay (RIA) is a technique that measures antigens by using antigens labeled with radioisotopes.

Rapid plasma regain (RPR) is a non-treponemal and non-specific test used in clinical laboratories to screen for syphilis, and it is the modified version of the

VDRL test where RPR antigen suspension contains choline chloride for greater stability, and charcoal to read the results without the need for a microscope.

Regulatory T (Treg) cells are one of CD4$^+$ T cell populations that express CD25 (IL-2 receptor α chain) and FoxP3 (transcription factor), the main function of Treg cells is to down-regulate other activated T cells and maintain peripheral tolerance to self-antigens.

RF latex agglutination test is an agglutination test that uses latex coated particles to detect RF in RA patients and it is a very useful tool in the follow-up of RA patients.

Rheumatic fever is caused by group A streptococcus-produced antibodies, which have cross-reactivity with the antigens of the heart, kidneys, and joints.

Rheumatoid arthritis (RA) is an autoimmune disease that affects the joints and causes inflammation of the joint.

Rheumatoid facter (RF) usually consists of IgM autoantibodies that are produced in RA to attack self-IgG.

RIA tracer is a radioactive labeled antigen used to compete with antigen (test antigen) in patient serum.

Ring precipitation is the precipitation of antibodies and antigens to form a desk between the top layer of the antigens and the bottom layer of the antibodies. The test is usually performed in a tube.

Sandwich ELISA uses an antibody specific to the patient target antigen and captures enzyme-labeled antibodies specific to the patient target antigen as well.

Secondary lymphoid organ is considered the home of mature T and B cells in which they proliferate and differentiate after recognizing their specific antigens.

Serology includes techniques that use antibodies to detect specific target antigens.

Serotyping serologically detected antigenic differences between infectious organisms.

Serum agglutination test (SAT) is mainly used to detect *Brucella* antibodies in patient serum. *Brucella* antibodies in patient sample react with *Brucella* test antigens forming agglutination.

Single diffusion is the diffusion of single particles, usually antigens, to form precipitin in agar medium containing specific antibodies.

Streptococcus pyogenes are Gram-positive bacteria, also known as group A streptococcus.

Streptolysin O (SLO) is an endotoxin produced by group A streptococcus that can lyse the host RBCs and white blood cells.

Super-antigens are antigens that activate all Vβ gene segment-expressing T cells.

Syphilis is a chronic bacterial infection caused by *Treponema pallidum* and transmitted sexually.

T cell receptors (TCRs) are expressed by T cells and are specific to certain antigens. TCRs consist of two regions: the variable (V) region that binds to antigens (antigen-binding site) and the constant (C) region, which is transmembranl.

T cells are lymphocytes that develop and mature in the thymus and are one of the adaptive immune cells.

T helper (Th) cells are T cells that express CD4 and interact with MHC class II expressed on the surface of APCs. Th cells are divided into five main subpopulations Th1, Th2, Th17, Th$_{Fh}$, and Tregs. Following the activation of each subpopulation, a different set of cytokines is produced that induces inflammation, supports B cell activation, or down-regulates the immune system.

Th1 is a CD4$^+$ T cell subset that mainly produces IL-2, IFN-γ, and TNF-α; they are involved in activating the cells of the immune system and supporting IgG$_3$ production by B cells.

Th17 is a CD4$^+$ T cell subset that mainly produces IL-17 and IL-22; they are involved in bacterial and fungal infections and autoimmunity.

Th2 is a CD4$^+$ T cell subset that mainly produces IL-4, IL-5, and IL-13; they are involved in parasitic and allergic responses.

Th$_{Fh}$ is a CD4$^+$ T cell subset that mainly supports B cell activation and differentiation.

Treponema palladium hemagglutination (TPHA) test is a specific hemagglutination treponemal test for syphilis that uses avian RBCs coated (sensitized) with *Treponema pallidum* antigens.

Treponemal test is a specific test for detecting syphilis and is used in clinical laboratories to confirm positive results obtained from a non-treponemal test.

Tube SAT provides the quantity of *Brucella* antibodies in patient serum following antibodies binding to *Brucella* antigens and the formation of an agglutination in the test tube.

Undulant fever is a bacterial infection caused by *B. abortus* and characterized by irregular episodes of fever.

Venereal disease research laboratory (VDRL) test see RPR.

Zoonotic describes an infection that is transmitted from animals to human.

Index

A

Active immunization, 6, 12
Active, passive and adoptive immunization,
    5–6
Acute phase proteins, 59
Adaptive, 1, 3–8, 12, 55
Adaptive immunity, 4–8
Adaptiveness, 6
Adoptive immunization, 6
Advantages, 23, 28, 31, 84
Advantages and limitations, 28, 31
Affinity, 18, 84
Agarose gel, 105, 107
Agarose gel electrophoresis, 112, 114
Agarose gel requirements and preparation, 112
Agglutination, 17, 23, 26–30, 36–39, 41,
    43–46, 48–53, 56–62, 81, 102
Ag stability, 16
Alternative, 3
Anamnestic response, 6
Antibodies, 4–7, 10–12, 15, 17–18, 23–31,
    34–36, 43, 44, 49, 50, 52, 63, 65, 74,
    75, 77, 78, 80, 81, 83, 84, 88, 90, 91,
    93, 94, 98, 103, 105, 107, 109, 112,
    119, 120, 122, 124–126
Antibodies & antigen interaction, 17–18
Antibody-mediated immunity, 42
Anti-citrullinated protein antibody (ACPA), 49
Antigen, 3–7, 12, 15, 17–18, 21–27, 29, 30, 32,
    34, 44, 53, 67–70, 72, 77, 78, 83, 84, 88,
    90, 91, 94, 112, 119, 122, 125, 126
Antigen and MHC molecules, 16
Antigen chemical complexity, 16
Antigen foreignness, 16
Antigen molecular weight, 16

Antigen-presenting cells (APCs), 3, 4, 6–8, 10,
    16, 21
Antigens, 15–16, 94
Anti-streptolysin O (ASO/ASL), 55
Application, 25, 26, 28, 29
The application of RF latex agglutination
    test, 50
Autoantibodies, 49, 52
Autoimmune, 1, 5, 26, 49, 52, 125
Autoreactive, 5
Avidity, 18, 27

B

Basophils, 2
B cell help, 8
B cell receptor (BCR), 5, 15
B cells, 4–13, 15, 17, 47, 49, 52, 55, 62
Biotinylated antigen, 88
Blood grouping, 29
B lymphocytes, 4
Brucella, 41
Brucella abortus, 41, 42
Brucella canis, 41
Brucella melitensis, 41, 42, 45
Brucella suis, 41, 42
Brucellosis, 41–43
Brucellosis incubation period, 43

C

C1q, 3
C2, 3
C3, 3, 11, 122, 124, 125
C4, 3

© Springer International Publishing AG, part of Springer Nature 2018
R. Y. Alhabbab, *Basic Serological Testing*, Techniques in Life Science and
Biomedicine for the Non-Expert, https://doi.org/10.1007/978-3-319-77694-1

$C_1V_1{=}C_2V_2$ method, 18
Cancer cells, 3
Capture antibodies, 84, 94
Cardiolipin, 31
CDC (Centers for Disease Control and
    Prevention), 43
$CD4^+$ T cells (T helper (Th) cells), 8
$CD8^+$ T cells (cytotoxic T (Tc) cells), 8
Cell mediated, 4, 8, 41
Cell-mediated immunity, 8
Cells involved in the adaptive immune system,
    6–7
Cells of the innate immune system, 2–3
Cell-surface virulence factors, 55
The cellular and the humoral adaptive immune
    system, 7–8
Cellular responses, 7
Cellulose acetate (cellogel) membrane
    electrophoresis, 113, 114
CFT reagents preparation, 64
Characteristics of the adaptive immune
    system, 6
Charcoal particles, 32
Chemical barriers, 1, 2, 10
Choline chloride, 32
Chronic inflammation, 1, 49
Classical, 3, 11
Clonal expansion, 1, 4
Clonally deleted cells, 5
Clonally expand, 4, 12
Clonal selection theory, 4–5
Competitive ELISA, 88, 91
Complement, 3–4
Complementary antibodies, 77, 78, 84
The complement C′ back titration, 69
Complement fixation test (CFT),
    63–74
Complement indirect immunofluorescence,
    124
Complement system, 1–4, 122, 125
Conjugate, 84, 88, 91, 98
Conjugated antibody, 119
Control line, 98
Corynebacterium diphtheriae, 26
Counts per minute (CPM), 80
C-reactive proteins (CRPs), 28, 59–62
Cross-reactivity, 33
CRP latex agglutination test, 60–61
C-type lectin receptors (CLRs), 3
Cytokine production, 8
Cytokines, 5, 8, 12, 59, 62, 97, 126
Cytotoxic cells, 3
Cytotoxic function, 8

D
Dendric cell (DCs), 2–4, 6, 10, 12
Densitometry, 113, 115
Developmental stages, 6
Diluent volume, 19
Dilution factor (DF), 18
Dilution factor method, 18–19
Dilutions, 18–20
Direct agglutination, 28
Direct ELISA, 83, 88
Direct IF, 119
Divalent, 18
Double immunofluorescence, 122

E
Electropherogram, 115
Electrostatic forces, 18, 22
ELISA reagents and steps, 88–91
ELISA results interpretation, 92–93
Endosome-lysosome mechanism, 55
Environmental control, 20
Enzyme immunoassay (EIA), 83
Enzyme-linked immunosorbent assay
    (ELISA), 34, 39, 48, 49, 59, 77, 81,
    83–95, 97, 102, 125
Eosinophils, 2, 10
Epitope, 5, 7, 17
Equivalence, 24, 105, 112
Example, 67

F
Fc receptors, 7
Fragment antigen binding (Fab), 7, 17, 18, 22
Fragment crystallizable (Fc), 7, 17, 22, 52, 84,
    90, 94, 122, 124
Freeze drying/lyophilization, 77

G
Gamma counter, 78
Gel diffusion precipitation test, 25
Glomerulonephritis, 55, 56
Granulocytes, 2
Group A streptococcus (GAS), 55, 56, 58
Grouping streptococci, 25

H
HCG one-step pregnancy urine test device,
    98–99
Hemagglutination, 28–29

Hemolysin, 65, 67
Hemolytic dose giving 50% lysic (HDSO), 67
HIV, 39
Homeostasis, 1
HsCRP, 59, 62
Human chorionic gonadotropin (hCG), 97
Humoral immunity, 7
Humoral responses, 4
Hydrophobic forces, 18

I
^{125}I, 77
IgA, 7, 17, 49, 105, 107, 112
IgD, 7, 17
IgE, 7, 17
IgG, 7, 17, 18, 35, 36, 38, 39, 49, 52, 78, 105, 107, 112, 116
IgM, 7, 17, 18, 35, 36, 38, 49, 105, 107, 109, 112
IL-1, 59, 62
IL-6, 59, 62
IL-10, 8, 62
Immunodiffusion, 26, 81, 105–107
Immunofixation electrophoresis (IFE), 111–118
Immunofluorescence (IF), 119–126
Immunofluorescence assay, 119–125
Immunogen, 15
Immunogenicity, 16
Immunoglobulin (Ig), 7, 17, 107
Immunoglobulin structure, 17
Immunoprecipitates, 112
Indirect ELISA, 84, 90
Indirect hemagglutination, 29, 36
Indirect IF, 120, 124
Indirect immunofluorescence complement fixation, 122
Inflammatory role, 8
Innate, 1–4, 8–11, 59
Innate immunity, 2–4
Interferon, 2
Intracellular gram-negative bacterium., 41
Ion exchange chromatography, 77

L
Lateral flow chromatographic immunoassay, 98
Latex, 26, 28, 49–51, 53, 56–62, 109
Latex reagent, 50, 56, 60
Leader, 112
Lectin, 3
Light chain amyloidosis (AL), 111
Lipopolysaccharide (LPS), 3, 41, 48

Loading dye, 112, 118
Lymphocyte-specific receptors, 5

M
Macrophage migration inhibitory factor, 97
Macrophages, 2, 3, 6, 8, 10, 41, 49, 55
Macroscopic, 31
Major histocompatibility complex (MHC), 6, 8, 12, 16
Malta fever, 42, 48
Mannan moieties, 3
Mediterranean fever, 42
Membrane attack complex (MAC), 3
Memory, 4, 6, 12
Monoclonal gammopathies (MG), 111
Monoclonal gammopathy of undetermined significance (MGUS), 111
Monocytes, 2, 3, 8
Mononucleosis, 51
The most pathogenic *Brucella* species to humans, 42
M protein, 111, 117
Multivalent Ag, 17
Mutation, 5

N
Natural killer (NK) cells, 2, 3, 12
Neutrophils, 2
NOD-like receptors (NLRs), 3
Non-phagocytic epithelial cells, 41
Non-specific binding (NSB), 78
Non-treponemal test, 31, 32

O
Opsonize, 3
Optimal sensitizing concentration (OSC), 67

P
Passive immunization, 6
Pathogen-associated molecular patterns (PAMPs), 3, 11, 55
Pattern recognition receptors (PRRs), 2, 3, 11, 55
Phagocytic cells, 2, 8, 10
Phagocytosis, 3, 7, 97
Phospholipid antigens, 31, 34
Physical and chemical barriers, 2
Physical barrier, 2
Plasma cells, 17

Platelets, 2, 10
Polymorphonuclear (PMN), 2
Positive control and antisera preparation, 70
Precipitation, 17, 22–26, 28, 30,
     109, 117
Precipitation technique, 24–26
Precipitin ring, 105, 107, 109
Preparation of complement and sensitized
     sRBCs, 65–67
Primary antibodies, 84, 90, 94
Primary chancre, 35
Principle, 24–29, 32, 36, 43–45, 50, 56,
     60–61, 63–64, 77–78, 83–88, 98, 105,
     112, 119–122
Progesterone, 97, 102

R
Radial immunodiffusion assay (RID),
     105–107
Radioimmunoassay (RIA), 77–81
Radioisotopes, 77
Rapid plasma reagin (RPR), 31–35, 39
Reagent pad, 98
Reagents, 44–46, 88, 90, 91, 98, 107,
     112–114, 122–125
Reagents and materials used, 50
Reagents provided in the kit, 64
Reagents that must be provided in the
     kit, 36
Regulatory function, 8
Regulatory immune cells, 5
Regulatory T (Tregs) cells, 5
Rejection, 97
Results example, 46
Results interpretation, 37–38, 51, 61, 72–74,
     99, 107, 115–116, 125
Results window, 98
RF latex agglutination, 50–51
RF latex agglutination test
     limitation, 51
RF latex agglutination test steps, 51
Rheumatic fever, 55, 56
Rheumatoid arthritis, 28, 49, 52, 53
Rheumatoid factor (RF), 49
RIA reagents, 78
RIA results interpretation, 80–81
RIA steps, 78–80
RID plate, 107
RIG-like receptors (RLRs), 3
Ring precipitation, 24–25
RPR test reagents, 32
RPR test steps, 33

S
Sample pad, 98
Sandwich ELISA, 84, 90–91
Screening, 31, 34
Second antibodies, 84
Secondary antibodies, 77, 78, 84, 94, 120
Secondary lymphoid organs, 3
Secondary phase, 27
Secondary stage, 35
Second plate, 69
Secreted virulence factors, 55
Semi-quantitative, 27, 36, 50, 56
Sensitivity, 49, 59, 77, 84, 97
Sensitized sheep RBCs, 64
Serial dilution, 19–20
Serological, xii, 15, 17, 18, 23, 31, 34, 42, 58
Serological tests to detect Brucellosis, 43
Serotyping, 17
Serum-agglutination test, tube (SAT), 44–46
Sexually transmitted, 31, 35
Single diffusion, 25–26
Slide agglutination test, 43–44
Specific, 6
Specimen window, 98
Standard, 64, 67–70, 78, 88, 90–92, 95
Standard antigen preparation, 67–70
Steps, 44, 88, 90, 91, 98, 107, 114–115
Streptococci group B toxins, 28
Streptococcus pyogenes, 55
Streptolysin O (SLO), 55
Super-antigens, 55
Syphilis, 31, 34, 35

T
T and B lymphocytes, 4
T cell receptor (TCR), 5, 16
T cells, 3–9, 11–13, 16, 47, 49
Tertiary infection, 35
T follicular helper (T$_{Fh}$), 8
Th1, 8, 13
Th17, 8, 49, 52
Th2, 8, 13
T line, 98
TLR-4, 3
TLR-9, 3, 11
TLRs, 3, 11
TNF-α, 59
Total binding (TB), 78, 80
Total count (TC), 78, 80, 81
Total volume, 19
Tracer, 78, 80
Transfer volume, 19

Treg, 8, 12
Treponemal test, 31, 35
Treponema pallidum, 31, 34, 35
Treponema pallidum hemagglutination
    (TPHA), 31, 34–39

U
Undulant fever, 42
Univalent, 17, 22

V
Van der Waals forces, 18
Venereal disease research laboratory (VDRL),
    31–35, 39
Viral hemagglutination, 28
Virally infected, 3

Z
Zoonotic, 41

Printed in the United States
By Bookmasters